**Campbell Armstrong** is the author of many novels including *Jig*, *Mambo* and *Mazurka*. He was born in Glasgow and in 1971 moved to America with his wife and three sons. In 1978 he started to write full time and in 1991, after twenty years in the US, he moved to Ireland where he now lives with his wife, Rebecca.

*Also by Campbell Armstrong*

# All That
# Really Matters

CAMPBELL ARMSTRONG

**WARNER BOOKS**

A *Warner* Book

First published in Great Britain in 2000
by Little, Brown and Company
This edition published by Warner Books in 2001

A CIP catalogue record for this book
is available from the British Library.

ISBN 0 7515 3079 4

Typeset in Horley OS by M Rules
Printed and bound in Great Britain by
Clays Ltd, St Ives plc

Warner Books
A Division of
Little, Brown and Company (UK)
Brettenham House
Lancaster Place
London WC2E 7EN

www.littlebrown.co.uk

*This book is dedicated to two remarkable souls,*
*Eileen and Barbara.*

# Acknowledgements

A deep debt of gratitude is due to the following people:

Imogen Taylor and Doug Pepper for their brave decisions, and editorial insights.

Thomas Congdon for his kindness and optimism, and for bearing with the project from start to finish.

Diana Tyler in London, and Richard Pine in New York, for their persistence.

Eileen's children – Stephen, who gave selflessly; Iain, who worked as hard as he knew how; Keiron, whose good heart helped us through. Barbara's children – Heidi and Mat and Marcus, who made this difficult journey with their mother, with understanding. This book couldn't have been written without them.

Sydney Altman, for his recollections and help.

Brenda Harris, for her help.

Eileen and Barbara's friends – too many to mention individually. They know who they are.

The wonderful workers in the Hospice movement. They are real stars.

The good people at the Armadillo Grill, in Phoenix, for their regular sustenance.

My wife Rebecca, for insisting that I should write this book, and for her encouragement through a difficult time.

And the late much-missed Nancy Frick, who provided a great deal of background material, and was always, always, a real friend.

# Prologue

I remember the beginning like this.

I'm at home, standing at the windows of my office on a June evening in Ireland, and I'm on idle, one of my favourite conditions. A sunny day, rare in the disappointing summer of 1997. My son Stephen, visiting from the United States, has gone downstairs to make a phone call: his mother Eileen, my ex-wife, had an appointment that morning with a doctor in Phoenix, Arizona. A cough has been worrying her, and she's decided to have an X-ray and checkup. Stephen wants to know the results. All day long he's been a little preoccupied. He's usually outgoing and cheerful, his humour nicely marbled with absurdity and nonsense and bursts of mimicry. But today he's slipped a gear or two.

Behind me, across the floor of my cluttered office, where files and papers and notebooks stand in tottering stacks, the windows overlook an expanse of green fields, sun gleams in the plum-coloured leaves of a giant copper beech. The landscape appears in green good health, vigorous and vibrant.

Rebecca, my wife, is trying to catch a horse, but the animal's playing games with her, waiting until she gets very close then twisting away from her, so that she has to stalk it again. And the process begins anew. It's frisky business, human and horse, patience pitted against mischief.

An idyll of a day. The peaceful heart of the bog, that part of Ireland named Umbilicus Hiberniae on ancient maps – and apart from Rebecca, not another human being in sight. The River Shannon is only ten miles away, but few tourists stray into our small corner of the country, and those that do are usually lost in the infamous maze of Irish backroads. Signposts around here are few, and sometimes unhelpful. I find this charming in its way, but it's a charm that often escapes the understanding of strangers who get trapped driving in maddening circles.

I can't hear Stephen's conversation from where I'm standing; the house is old and big, and he's a long way off below in the kitchen.

Again I watch Rebecca and the horse from the window. I remember when she came to Ireland to look at the house I'd bought. The expression of stunned amazement on her face; *have you ANY idea how much work this place needs? Do you know what you've done, Campbell?* No, I had no idea. I wasn't practical. We moved in, aptly perhaps, on Halloween 1991, and endured a miserable winter with no heat, and rain pouring through the ceilings. Now, six years of restoration later, Rebecca has told me several times she wouldn't live anywhere else; she's come to love this house.

I have the feeling I should be working, perhaps making notes for a novel in progress, or jotting down ideas: the activities Rebecca calls 'pencil-sharpening'. In fact, I'm thinking about my son and his phone call to his mother. I have no reason to suppose there's anything wrong with Eileen. The last time we spoke she hadn't mentioned her health. She'd been more concerned with mine than her own.

I'd just been diagnosed as diabetic, an ailment that was a total mystery to me, and an affront of sorts, the way unwelcome surprises are. Diabetic? Me? It doesn't even run in our family! The symptoms had been fierce thirst and serious weight-loss and a general lassitude. Rebecca had been the first to mention the possibility of diabetes, which I dismissed at once. When I had it confirmed by a doctor that she was correct in her suspicion – her suspicions are usually all too correct – I immediately began to gather information on this disease that had zapped me out of the blue. One of the first things I did was to call Eileen and ask if she had any knowledge of the subject.

Now I notice on my desk the twenty-page fax she sent me on 19 May, just two months ago. It bears the logo of the health clinic in Phoenix where she works. At the beginning of the fax, which is a lengthy extract from a medical journal explaining diabetes and treatment and dietary measures, is a handwritten note in which she tells me she's arranged for me to phone one of the physicians at her clinic if I want further advice. She finishes her note with the words: *Campbell, I have a lot of people on your case.* This is typical of her. I imagine how she leaped into action, making phone calls, arranging photocopies of relevant articles. The sicknesses that afflict other people are her private enemies, and she fights them daily. Her battleground is a rough one. She's a dedicated warrior, though, and an energetic survivor.

I hear Stephen on the stairs. I go to the doorway and watch him ascend. His expression is inscrutable. He reaches the landing and looks at me earnestly. He doesn't say anything for a time. When he finally speaks his voice is lifeless. I hear him talk but I don't absorb what he's telling me, and I ask him to repeat it. He does. And just for a moment something about him – his eyes, or the shape of his face – reminds me of Eileen when she was young.

# 1

I think of Glasgow, 1961, a crossroads in my young life: the year I dropped out of school because I wanted to write, but more important the year I met Eileen. I needed 'experience' of what I thought was the real world because how else would I have anything to write about? Specifically I wanted to write about my native city, which I found brooding and sinister, a place where skies were always grey and shadows gloomier than anywhere else. This wasn't the city that twenty-something years later would be zealously cleaned and sand-blasted and restored to its ornate Victorian-merchant splendour – no, in the early 60s this was a big grubby town of a million people, its streets traversed by tramcars, shaky double-decker cousins of American trolleys, whose electric overhead wires would short and spark and flash now and then like fireworks in the rain – it was always raining in Glasgow, and if it wasn't raining it was smoky, and the air sometimes so thick and foul with coal soot you might have been living through an eclipse. This wasn't the Glasgow that would later be brutalised by an expressway running directly through its heart like a sharp stake, where soulful old pubs would be transformed into theme bars, and fancy restaurants proliferate and fast-food joints multiply; where there would be shopping malls haunted by kids in high-tech sneakers, a fashionable Italian Centre, and expensive apartments in formerly dead areas of the city.

It was a vibrant, friendly, hard-bitten blue-collar city whose main industry, shipbuilding, was in decline. The big vessels of the world were being built elsewhere, in places where labour was cheaper and industrial disputes happened with less frequency. Glasgow has always had a Red history – my own grandfather, James Campbell, had been something of a socialist agitator on the River Clyde, a soapbox orator.

I'd been born a few streets from the river. My earliest memories were of the booming sounds from busy shipyards and the astringent oily smell of the small grimy tugboat that ferried people from one bank of the narrow river to the other. The Govan Ferry, it was called. The trip took all of a minute, sixty seconds of thick petrol smoke and the hysteria of disturbed gulls and the painful deafening throb of the engine. The Clyde was in my blood, in my imagination.

This was my city. This was the place I'd write about. I began to plan a Major Novel structured along the lines of Dos Passos' *USA* trilogy – contrapuntal was the really fancy word for it. Ah, Jesus, the *soaring* self-belief and innocence of youth, of a life without limitations. The book would be written in a style that owed much to Dylan Thomas, whose florid prose enchanted me. I was under the influence in those days. I was drowning in influences. Camus. Sartre. Dos Passos. Kerouac. My fellow Scot Robert Louis Stevenson. Who needed a leaving certificate anyway – even if quitting school meant separation from a wonderful English teacher called

Walter Wyatt, a man of great learning and infinite patience and the ability to bring to life the works of Chaucer and Wordsworth on squid-black Glasgow afternoons?

As I planned the Big Novel I was exploring the city. There was no significant after-hours nightlife in those years – bars were shut promptly at nine-thirty PM. On Sundays you couldn't find alcohol except in a hotel, and even then you had to be a hotel resident or a 'bona fide traveller' – a weird concept loosely defined as somebody who was able to prove they'd journeyed a specific number of miles if they wanted to be served booze; a Presbyterian bit of lunacy in the law, but people walked in great thirsty processions on Sundays to hotels that lay on the city limits.

Drinking in Glasgow back then was zoo-like. People pawed one another and fought in scrums for that last pint of beer on the ale-swamped counter before the awful closing-time bell. But drinking, everybody knew, was essential to the writer's development and self-image. What writer worth a damn didn't have a penchant for the lowlife? So I favoured pubs in mean streets – places I romanticised, places that would have horrified my parents, who were already disappointed with me for leaving school a month before getting a Certificate of Higher Education, or whatever the paper was called. I wanted to capture the 'patter', the rhythms and colloquialisms of Glasgow speech. I enjoyed pubs where you met characters, old prizefighters and their corner men, bookies, rummies, petty criminals, low-grade con artists, gangsters and thugs, warned-off jockeys, and the occasional football player whose career always seemed to have been interrupted by the Second World War.

Memories of a war that had finished sixteen years before lingered in Glasgow; the Luftwaffe had attacked the ship-yards, and bombs had fallen all over the city. There were still bomb shelters behind tenements, frail brick things that looked like they couldn't stop a bullet, let alone powerful German explosives dropped from thousands of feet. Many of the shelters were ruined smelly places where tramps – 'dossers' in the local patois – slept, or where drunks went when the pubs were shut, where cats pissed and dogs shit, and where sometimes people, too impassioned or inebriated to care about their surroundings, screwed. There were also scores of vacant lots where tenements, struck by German warplanes, had once stood.

You almost never met women in the bars I frequented, masculine sanctuaries always dimly lit, where men spat and swore and invariably smoked the harsh ill-named Woodbine. The preferred drink was a vicious apple extract called scrumpy that had the effect of dismantling your perceptions utterly. And if scrumpy wasn't available there was a cheap wine called VP actually *brewed* in Glasgow (could there be, I wondered, a mysterious vineyard tucked away in a private pocket of Tuscan sunlight in a mythical part of the city known only to a few?). Alas, VP was actually concocted in a factory in the East End and processed in vats where rodents were said to drown. The initials, some alleged, stood for Vat Piss, sometimes Vat Pus. The stuff, sweet and red and unpalatable, was guaranteed to cause brief hallucinations of a poetic type, followed by sapping hangovers the next day.

I was still officially living with my parents in the extreme eastern part of the city where new housing estates flourished – we'd moved from the friendly old tenement culture of the city's south side on my seventh birthday to this isolated gulag of new houses, each with its own balcony or 'verandah' – but I was spending many nights sleeping on the floors or sofas in friends' houses. The novel wasn't progressing in terms of words on paper. I didn't even own a typewriter. I didn't own any paper either. I convinced myself I was note-taking in my head; I was 'storing' impressions for some future date – which was all very well up to a point, but it wasn't providing me with income.

I needed some kind of job. It didn't much matter what it was.

My mother slipped me money from time to time, especially when my father wasn't looking, but that couldn't continue. She was an easy touch, with a heart as big as the city itself; her generosity made me guilty. Father was a little aloof at times, detached. He was a good father, he provided for his family without fail, he was never out of work, he drank only in mod-eration, he didn't beat his wife (on the contrary, he served her breakfast in bed every Sunday of their marriage); he neither encouraged nor discouraged his son's ambitions, so he could never be accused of standing in anyone's way – but there was always a sense of distance between us. In later years, I won-dered if this was due to the fact that when he came home from the war in late 1945 I was already one year old and had usurped him to some degree in my mother's attentions, and consequently a mild bacterial strain of resentment persisted. I was never sure; it wasn't the kind of question you asked him. He rarely spoke of himself or his feelings: he was a product of a generation that didn't acknowledge the value of self-explo-ration. Examining your life? Waste of time.

Both parents worked. We were, I suppose, working-class comfortable. My father was employed by the Harland & Wolf shipyard, my mother – who had an amazing knack for mental arithmetic – was a book-keeper. There was no memory of anyone else in the family with the ambition to be a writer, no genetic forerunner. It was some kind of oddity, although to me it was perfectly natural. I can pinpoint the precise moment

when I came to the decision, or at least had it thrust upon me:
a six-year-old's epiphany. I was listening absent-mindedly to
the radio and I heard a man reading a poem called *And Death
Shall Have No Dominion*. The reader was Dylan Thomas and
I can recall with great clarity the big over-dramatic voice and
the sounds of the words, as surely as I can see the coal fire
burning in the kitchen grate and a navy-blue winter afternoon
pressing against the windowpanes.

The meaning of the poem was years beyond me, but the
*words* – the words rolled and vibrated through me, they
thrilled; 'dominion' – which I'd never heard before – conjured
up for some reason faraway foreign places, Spanish vistas, blue
seas, treasure, magic. Who can say where that stuff came
from? In what fissure of the brain an unknown word found
resonance? I thought: *I want to work in words*. In a small boy's
head a decision had been made, and nothing would change it.
I wrote all through primary school – poems, short stories;
through high school, journalism, essays, it didn't matter the
form, I enjoyed the act of writing. Making things up, forcing
pictures into words, setting words on paper, taking pleasure
even in so small a matter as the shapes of certain letters and
how they looked when they were placed alongside others.

So I was a trainee engineer of language, terrific – but there
was still no income. The major drawback of the unpublished
writer's life: you need a day job. I had left school without a
diploma. I wasn't qualified for anything that demanded special
skills. I wasn't exactly fascinated by the prospect of the day-
to-dayness of an ordinary job in any case – but it was a fate I
couldn't avoid. So I found work in a store called Cuthbertson's
on Glasgow's most famous shopping thoroughfare,
Sauchiehall Street, an old-fashioned establishment that sold
sheet music, pianos and other musical instruments on the
upper floors, and record albums in the basement.

I was assigned to the basement. In that overheated cellar, where ventilation was nonexistent and the air smelled of trapped cigarette smoke, my future was about to take shape among the listening-booths and the racks of the latest long-playing releases and the cardboard cut-out PR displays of smiling popular singers. Because it was here that Eileen worked – a swivel of fate I couldn't sidestep, one with life-altering consequences.

I was the only full-time male on the staff in the lower depths. The other five employees were all women whose ages ranged from about nineteen to thirty. For the first time in my life I was privy to the private conversations of women, their secrets, stories of their love affairs, the aspirations of their hearts, their ambitions and daydreams and disappointments. In the staffroom at the back of the basement – little more than a dusty cobwebbed boiler-room with a table and a couple of chairs and an electric kettle – they took their breaks and conducted their inquests on failed relationships or discussed a specific customer who'd set their heartbeat racing. They appeared to be unconscious of my maleness. They talked in front of me as if I were either the inoffensive idiot brother or an item of forgotten furniture, it didn't matter which: I was a harmless fixture either way.

I could sit and watch as they applied makeup, or brushed their hair, or adjusted items of clothing, such as the garter- or suspender-belt, which has become almost extinct. The realignment of this device involved the woman standing up and turning away in a manner both coy and absent-minded, hitching up her skirt quickly, then a hidden motion of the hand followed by a quick smoothing down of the skirt, and resumption of normal behaviour. I could observe them at such chores as plucking eyebrows, mirrors perched close to their faces, tweezers poised. Or the application of nail varnish, which was a drawn-out process involving not only the delicate movement of a small glossy wet brush but also the drying time and the pungent scent of chemicals the women appeared never to notice. These rituals, these intimacies – I might have been studying the private rites of a tribe or the members of a masonic club. There was a sense in which it was a kind of privilege: I could eavesdrop to my heart's content. Sometimes I was even invited to talk.

'You're a man, Campbell. Do you think Rosemary should go out with that bloke who wears the blue duffel coat?'

Or: 'Do you think women should be pushy, Campbell? Do you think Kathy should just come on to a guy she likes? Do you think the guy will respect her for being forward? What's your opinion, Campbell? Eh? Tell us.'

I believe they only asked these questions to make me feel I was an acceptable adjunct to the tribe, if not a full member. At other times I had a suspicion they were playing a game at my expense, I was the only male, therefore outgunned and easily outsmarted – the questions were trick questions, I wasn't really expected to answer them. I was being set up for something, albeit in the nicest way. Sometimes I was teased – *Hey, Campbell, tell us about your love life, you hear all about ours. Give us the intimate details, come on, come on, hold nothing back, we're all ears. Don't spare us. We're big girls, we can take it. You're no' a monk, are you?*

The dry Glasgow sense of humour, developed in the streets and workplaces and refined in the old music-halls, always depended on a deadpan delivery, sometimes to the extent that you couldn't tell a joke from a serious comment. It was banter, quick and sly, that ruled in the basement.

Officially, Eileen was assistant manager of the record department. She was around twenty-three, about five years older than me. Usually she was the last person to appear in the morning – arriving flustered, handbag open, coat flapping, no makeup, cigarette in hand, some wild story to tell. She hadn't been to bed until four AM. She had a whale of a hangover. She'd mixed her booze badly last night. She'd met some guy and gone on to a party. Her life seemed vibrantly haphazard to me. She was lively, scattered, funny, forever on the edge of some great upheaval or other – a potential boyfriend, perhaps a new job offer, a flat she was planning to rent but couldn't decide if she wanted it or if she could afford it. (We were seriously – *scandalously* – underpaid in the basement.) It always struck me that in reality she didn't give a damn one way or the other about these little dramas. Life for her was something you lived, and if you couldn't laugh about it, if you couldn't throw yourself in at the deep end, then you didn't deserve it.

She'd dump the contents of her purse on the table in the staffroom – cosmetic paraphernalia, busted cigarettes, ticket stubs, tampons, mismatched earrings – and then she'd start to make herself presentable for the day's work. This was always a complex operation, but she had it down to a fast art. It was like watching a speeded-up movie. She'd brush her red hair, which she wore short at this time, in broad strokes. She'd take a couple of puffs on a cigarette without losing the fluency of her movement. The lipstick (usually a bright pink or something similar). Some kind of powder (always just a touch). Eyeliner (sparing). Mascara (even more sparing). A few more drags on her cigarette, a couple of slugs of coffee, and she'd be transformed from an AM wreck into somebody fetchingly presentable, ready to deal with the day's customers. She always wore bright colours, and if they clashed – what the hell, it didn't matter.

She was just over five feet tall. Her face was oval, and she had a tiny gap between her front teeth. She wasn't beautiful in any traditional sense of that word, but she had a delightful air of mischief about her, an impish quality, and a smart, sharp light in her eyes. As a child, she'd wanted to become a ballerina. She liked to dance still, even if the ambition had long since dissolved. She didn't have the classic ballet dancer's shape; her breasts were too big for the slender androgynous look, the ideal.

Her education wasn't extensive. It had ended at secretarial college level where she'd learned basic office skills: I couldn't imagine her being happy taking dictation and filing flimsy copies of letters she'd typed. She wasn't bookish. She wouldn't have made it in the academic world. She enjoyed working in the record department because she liked music, the responsibility of deciding which albums to buy, and trading barbs with the record company reps – comedians for the most part, fast-talking salesmen. Her knowledge of music was wide.

I sometimes had the vague impression, for no specific reason, that she didn't have half the confidence she tried to project, that under the seemingly blunderbuss approach she took to life, the haphazard exterior and all the easy repartee with salesmen, she wasn't exactly imbued with self-assurance: something troubled her, something gnawed at her on a level she didn't want to explore. What did I see there? A sadness? A slight haunting? A hidden fragility? Or was I inventing a mysterious persona for her? I wasn't sure.

We began to spend time together. It was innocent, sharing tea in the staffroom, or sandwiches or quickly heated canned spaghetti at lunch. I liked her, I knew that. I was intrigued by the currents of her life, stories of her mishaps. There was a Keystone Kop element to her misadventures. They always involved the wrong train, the wrong bus, a taxi to the wrong address. She had a stand-up's sense of timing and a good line in self-derision. She disliked pomposity, people with affectations. If she had plans and ambitions, she didn't speak about them. I felt she was just going with the flow, years before that phrase entered our language.

She encouraged me to tell her about my writing (I was out of the Big Novel for the time being and into the heavyweight poetic stage) and she listened sympathetically. I felt free to talk; she gave me the opportunity to ventilate pressures that had been building up in my head. I could speak to her about anything, books I wanted to write, poems. She was never judgmental. There was no ridicule, no mockery. She never derided my dreams. I often gave her my poems to read and she always returned them with a favourable comment or two. I look at some of these poems today with embarrassment. How trite they are, how wilfully obscure. I can't decipher them. I wonder what she really thought of them. All I remember is that she was generous with her time, and sympathetic, even if I must have seemed like a geyser of words to her, a wild-eyed intense young man, often hungover, ranting. It didn't matter – she always had the graceful knack of listening.

We were becoming friends, but I was still no part of her world away from work. She seemed to attend a lot of parties, she knew where good music could be heard (she usually had tickets for big events), she knew where the late-night clubs were located (a subterranean aspect of Glasgow in those days), she always seemed to have men in pursuit of her, and sometimes she had to juggle them. I learned that despite her hectic social life, she still lived with her parents in the relatively prosperous genteel southern suburb of Giffnock, she slept in the same bedroom she'd had as a young child, and she had a dog called Rebel – tiny details, the borders of somebody's life, nothing of substance.

I also learned she was Jewish. This was a touch of unexpected exotica. Even though I'd known there was a small Jewish community in Glasgow, I'd never run into anyone Jewish before. It wasn't by choice, it just hadn't happened. Glasgow was polarised along religious lines, Protestants on one side, Catholics on the other, a city of tiresome and tragic segregation: Jews, though, were beyond this divide. They formed a small third tribe that existed, largely ignored, outside the two bigger ones. I knew absolutely nothing about Jewish life and customs beyond the fact that Jews didn't eat pig. Eileen explained a few basics to me: she wasn't allowed to have a non-Jewish boyfriend and most certainly *not* a non-Jewish husband (a statement delivered with a look of *oh-yeah* scepticism); her mother kept a strict kosher household and separated the meat and dairy dishes (a practice Eileen thought tedious); meat had to be bought from a kosher butcher and then salted to drain it of blood (another tradition for which she had no affection: koshering meat deprived it of taste – *what a waste of a decent steak*). She ignored these taboos. Her rebellion against religious customs struck me as part of some greater form of revolt – against the conventions of the times, and the strictures of Glasgow, which still felt as if it were run by a stern committee of church elders. She was looking for fun. She was looking to kick away the struts of propriety. She didn't want to live in a world of dead Sundays and nights that perished drably after nine-thirty.

As she and I grew closer over a period of four or five months, and our friendship strengthened, I had the feeling at times that her relationship with me – which was moving ineluctably towards something beyond platonic – was another way she'd found of flaunting acceptable standards. Not only was I *not* Jewish, I was five years *younger* than her, and in the framework of the times it was OK for the woman to be five years younger than the man, but very unusual and not entirely *correct*, God knows why, for the roles to be reversed.

So we began to meet after work. We'd have drinks in one or other of the various bars around the city centre, or if she had tickets to a concert, which she received *gratis* from record-company salesmen or promoters, we'd go listen to music – often jazz, often one of the legends who flew into Glasgow: Gerry Mulligan, Stan Getz, Chet Baker. Neither of us knew where this relationship was headed; it was enough for the present that we found pleasure in each other's company. There was no future, nor any talk of one. Sometimes I'd ride a bus to the south side of the city close to where she lived and we'd meet – always at a safe distance from her parents' house – and we'd walk together through a wooded area alongside an old railtrack, or we'd go further south to a park called Rouken Glen where a waterfall roared down into a terraced glade, one of her favourite spots, sweet and green and shaded.

To use a quaint phrase, we were actually *courting*, we were stepping out together. Dating. This sneaked up on us, took us unawares. She couldn't possibly tell her parents about me. The wrath of her mother, Doris, was seemingly the last thing she wanted to incur. She used expressions such as *I don't want to let my mother down* and *I don't want to disappoint her*. As for her father, Israel, apparently an easygoing man, she was determined not to bring him any pain. There was almost an element of desperation in the way she wanted to protect her parents. From me? Nobody had ever needed protection from *me* before.

I assumed it was more on account of my gentile background than any age difference. No matter, nothing mattered, I was moving into that dizzy phase when the heart begins its countdown to lift-off and life has no limits, and everything is possible.

But we had a logistical problem to solve. We had nowhere to go. Absurd. She lived at home, and so did I, nominally at least. Hotels cost more than either of us could afford on the pittance paid by the music store. Besides, there was a dearth of affordable motels in the city at this time.

We had to get away somehow.

I don't remember whether she suggested it, or I did, but we decided on an overnight camping trip to the Campsies, a lovely range of hills about twelve miles from the city. Eileen said she liked the outdoors; for myself, I had no great fondness for tents and I was uneasy with the vicissitudes of Scottish weather, but at least we would have privacy, intimacy. We rode the bus to the foothills, and then walked a couple of miles until we found a location a few hundred yards from the road. We had a picnic basket, wine, a sleeping-bag, a couple of candles, and a flashlight with a weak battery. The night air smelled of rain. I soon had the tent in place; I was usually hopeless when it came to putting up tents but on this night, rapidly darkening and filled with promise, I got the structure in place and pegged securely down. After all – what intricacy is involved in setting up a two-man tent if you're a young man, impassioned and impatient?

Inside, we laid the sleeping-bag across the groundsheet and closed the flap of the tent and lit one of the candles and for a long time listened to the wind and the sound of cattle in a nearby field. We made small talk. Rain began to blow up. Candlelight flooded the green canvas interior, stamping huge shadows on the walls. We lay down together and listened to the weather flutter the tiny tent. We were isolated. The city was miles away. I felt . . . shy, perhaps. I was young, and this was the brink of love, and Eileen was a woman by contrast to the girls I'd known at school. I understood that whatever was taking place in this fragile wind-rattled shelter on a hillside was more than an uncomplicated sexual transaction; somehow, it was going to constitute a commitment.

Somehow it was going to lead into the future.

She had a scar an inch or so below her navel. By candlelight, I thought at first it was just a shadow. But no, it was a scar, slightly puckered, and I touched it with my fingertips. She covered my hand with her own: her eyes were wet. She looked sad and serious, an expression on her face I'd never seen before. I wondered about the scar – what was it? an appendectomy? It was surely a surgical trace of some kind. And it upset her, and not just because of any vanity.

She told me: it was a Caesarean scar.

'A Caesarean?' I asked.

'I had a baby. I ought to tell you that.'

I imagined a knife going into her flesh and shuddered. Skin peeled back, and blood, and the sudden emergence of a child.

'Where is the baby?' I asked.

She was overwhelmed, as if the word 'baby' had suddenly thrown open windows long shuttered, and light was flooding into rooms that had been locked for years. This was a memory she'd buried, small bones she didn't want disturbed.

I held her for a time and she cried, and in the hushed moments between tears she told me the story of her baby.

# 2

In 1954, when she was sixteen, she met a man eleven years older than she was. She never gave me any details about how she'd met him. His name was Bill. No job, no last name, and I didn't ask. She thought she loved him. She was, as she put it, very young and innocent, and her parents had known nothing about this relationship, which lasted for the better part of a year. I imagined it as she spoke – concealment, clandestine meetings: it had a familiar ring. I couldn't help but note its similarities to my own relationship with her.

I watched her by the light of the candle and wondered if she and Bill had gone to the same parks and taken the same walks and sat in the same cinemas as we did; was I following in the steps of this past love? She'd had to conceal Bill from her parents because of the age difference, whether he was Jewish or not (she never said if he was: he remains a shadowy mystery to this day, faded and lost). She couldn't introduce Doris and Issy to a man eleven years her senior – a cradle snatcher, for God's sake – any more than she could take home a kid like me.

Did she make a habit of choosing relationships with built-in difficulties, or were they just the kind of things she stumbled into because she followed her heart with no thought of consequences? This line of inquiry was beside the point. She was a romantic, and so was I, and we were together in a frail tent on a rainy hillside with our wine, and she was telling me the secret history of her life – we were falling in love, and that was when you shared the stuff of your past. I don't remember now any extreme jealousy or insecurity when I learned about Bill, although there must have been a flutter. But the matter was history and immutable, and besides, it was the idea of the baby that stunned and intrigued me.

When Eileen became pregnant, she knew very little about her body: apparently sex education wasn't the kind of topic Doris discussed around the house. She once told Eileen, in a piece of misinformation that might have made an old nun proud, that babies grew in the back yard. (In pea pods? The rhubarb patch? Dangling from a tomato trellis?) And then, in this household of biological myths and social respectability and basic decency, Eileen had the searing, unenviable task of announcing she was pregnant. There was no possibility of a mistake. She'd been to a physician and he'd confirmed her condition. She didn't have the courage to face her parents when it came right down to it, so she asked her favourite aunt and confidante, Aunt D, to tell Doris and Issy the story.

Eileen waited upstairs in her bedroom while Aunt D broke the news. Her state of mind, understandably, was one of extreme agitation. She wanted to jump out of the window – her bedroom was on the second floor – but she wasn't sure if the fall would be long enough to finish her life or simply maim her. She told me that this time was the worst in her life.

How would her parents react? She couldn't imagine looking her father in the face ever again. She was his little girl, his special girl. And her mother, a touch tightly strung at the best of times – Doris's response was easy to predict. Outrage, distress, anger, how could there be anything else? I pictured Eileen waiting, hands clenched in tension, thinking her young life ruined, perhaps hearing the indistinct rumble of voices from the living-room downstairs where Aunt D was revealing the unavoidable truth.

Eileen heard her mother crying loudly, hysterically. She went downstairs. It must have been the longest walk she'd ever taken. Doris confronted her. Words like 'disgrace' and 'scandal' and 'shame' crackled in the room like electrical disturbances. Her father, quiet and pale, was trying to comfort his wife. Aunt D was soothing, a truce-maker who brought the temperature down.

The inventive capacity of humans under stress can be breathtaking: a plan was concocted hurriedly. Since abortion was illegal, it wasn't even a consideration. It was an activity associated with backstreet butchers, the squalor of struck-off doctors performing terminations in unhygienic surroundings or seedy ex-nurses equipped with long rubber tubes, buckets of blood on mildewed rugs or cracked linoleum, knives and wire coathangers. It had dreadful connotations. The plan dreamed up by Doris and Issy involved a serious upheaval in their usually placid home life, and the weaving of an elaborate fiction that seems more complex than the unadorned truth would have been. But this was 1954 and the idea of a single mother carried the heavy burden of social stigma. The fallen woman, the bastard child. In Issy and Doris's world, the only feasible solution to Eileen's predicament was evasion.

This was the scheme they hatched: Israel would give up his furrier's business in Glasgow and they'd go to Scarborough, a coastal resort town in Yorkshire where they'd often vacationed. Among family and friends they'd circulate the story that Doris was suffering from a bad case of nerves, and needed 'rest' in a place removed from stress. She was following the fictional orders of a fictional doctor. She was willing to accept the indignity of the label 'nervous breakdown' rather than admit to anyone that her daughter was pregnant. Only one condition was imposed: in return for the support and care of her parents, Eileen would give the baby up for adoption.

No other choice, no argument, no room for bargaining. Doris was adamant. Forget. You have your whole life ahead of you. Adoption struck Eileen as a better solution than abortion, and she went along with it. Besides, she was grateful that her parents hadn't abandoned her. Quite the opposite, they were making sacrifices in their lives to support her. She knew that Israel's business hadn't been prospering, and that he couldn't really afford the cost of renting a house for months in Scarborough.

When the ordeal was over they'd all return to Glasgow and pick up the frayed threads of their interrupted lives, and nobody would ever think of the baby again. It would be one of those dark secrets families keep locked away, like old photographs stashed in a mildewed steamer-trunk in an attic. Apart from Aunt D, the only other person privy to the conspiracy was Eileen's brother Sydney, ten years older than she, who'd go to any lengths to protect the family name.

And he did, he kept the silence for years, until it was nothing more than a foggy memory.

In January 1955, Eileen and her parents travelled by bus to Scarborough, The town presented a bleak face to the North Sea that washed its sandy beaches. The familiar summer attractions – seafront shops selling fish and chips and whelks and candyfloss and breezy postcards and silly hats with suggestive slogans – were shuttered and lifeless. A holiday town in winter: nothing in the geography of England can be quite so bleak and cheerless. The seascape, dark and unpredictable, mirrored the mood of the family.

In Scarborough they settled into a rented house. Eileen spent time taking long walks, often in her father's company, on the promenade overlooking the wind-roughened sea, or along the beach. As she told me the story, I pictured the wind blowing in off wet sands and the tang of brine so sharp it stung your lungs, and Eileen huddled in a heavy coat, her face half-wrapped in a scarf. I saw her with her arm linked through her father's. An ordinary image – father and daughter walking together – but an extraordinary situation.

Neither Issy nor Doris ever asked questions about the baby's father. They just didn't want to know. It was as if they preferred to believe in immaculate conception. They created quite an impressive make-believe world in Scarborough, and in this fairytale place, this time out of time, anything could be suspended or ignored – even Doris's kosher discipline. When Eileen developed a craving for bacon sandwiches, Doris gave her the money to buy them. What did it matter? The real world was on hold. Eat what you like. This is a side-trip from reality. This is Fantasyland. Even the job Issy was obligated to take to provide the family's support – their rent was high, £3 a week – bore no relation to anything he'd done before. He became a milkman. It was a descent for him; after all, he'd had his own business. But now he rose in the miserable stinging blackness of wintry mornings to deliver bottles of milk.

Eileen began to think more and more of the child growing inside her. She was developing the proprietorial affection of a mother for her unborn baby. One day she asked Doris the unthinkable: might she keep the child? Doris told her to put that notion out of her head immediately.

Eileen said, 'It isn't right to give my baby away.'

'It's a hard thing to do, I know,' Doris said. 'But you won't regret it.'

Eileen didn't raise the matter again.

There was a piano in one room of the house. She didn't know how to play it but spent hour after hour there, picking out tunes, quietly singing lullabies to the unborn baby – *Hush Little Baby, Don't You Cry* was her favourite – forging a profound private bond she knew was going to be fruitless, unless Doris had an improbable change of heart.

This girl, ill-schooled in the intricacies of her body, was looking down the scary tunnel of birth, a journey into the unknown she'd never planned to take. She asked her mother questions – what will I feel? how long will it take? will I bleed? – and Doris, uncomfortable with this kind of talk, arranged for her to have prenatal care. If Eileen had questions, they might as well be answered by people who were experts in maternity.

Eileen couldn't help it, she kept coming back to the idea of keeping the baby. She'd find a way to do it. She'd get a job, she'd manage it all somehow. It wouldn't matter what anyone else thought. Her life was her own. Who had any right to take her child away from her? She entered a phase of quiet defiance, but she couldn't tell how deep her reserves of bravado might be.

When she was admitted to hospital, physicians discovered that the baby was lying in breech position, and that delivery could be achieved only through Caesarean section. On 30 May 1955, she gave birth to a healthy baby girl she named Barbara, after her favourite childhood doll. The idea of a girl having a baby she named after a childhood doll touched me when she told me: I thought of her in 1955 suspended in that spooky place between adolescence and adulthood, neither one thing nor the other, a child-woman.

She remained in hospital for three weeks to recover from surgery, and during this time she bottle-fed Barbara because she'd been given medication to dry her breast milk. Daily contact with a baby you have no chance of taking home and raising. You hold the child, kiss it, adore it, take it into your heart. Only you don't get to take it home. Such torture. The bond that had formed between Eileen and her baby during pregnancy was only strengthened by the intimacy of these daily encounters. How could she be forced to give this child away now?

Doris and Issy visited while she convalesced. Doris had developed a fiction for general distribution in the ward – her daughter's husband was a soldier stationed in Germany and couldn't be with his wife at present. Eileen went along with this fable: what was one more story when there had been so many already? Perhaps she even liked the idea of an absent soldier husband, a uniformed young man on patriotic duty.

During one visit, she asked Doris to bring a camera into the ward so that she might at least take a photograph of Barbara. But Doris didn't allow it on the grounds that photographs would only be upsetting later. No camera. Eileen waited until she was alone with the baby and laid her on the bed and lovingly traced the contours of the infant's face and body with her eye: if she couldn't have a physical photograph, she'd have a mental one at least, a picture she could look at whenever she wanted.

After three weeks, she was released from hospital. She now had a grace period – if grace is the word – of three more weeks in which to make her final decision about Barbara's future. The idea that this decision was Eileen's was another strand in the fiction: the decision had *always* been Doris's. At the end of three weeks, Eileen would appear at the offices of the adoption society where she'd be obliged to give up the child or keep her. Three weeks of anguish. She still nurtured the hope – slender as it was – that her mother might relent.

She went to the adoption society at the appointed time, where she was left alone with the baby for a short period. She held the child in her arms. She cried, pressing her damp face against the baby's. She wished there was another door through which she might escape, taking Barbara with her, disappearing into a place where they'd never be found.

To keep the child or to give her away? All Eileen's instincts inclined towards the former. But she knew she couldn't fight Doris on this one. A bargain had been struck and she couldn't go back on it now, unless Doris said so. When her parents re-entered the room, accompanied by social workers, Eileen turned to look at her mother imploringly. A last chance, a last-second reprieve, please. There was always a possibility, wasn't there?

No. One look at the expression on Doris's face killed any such chance. *It's done with. Get rid of the baby. Let's go home. I'm sorry it has to be this way.* In the most heart-breaking moment she had ever known, Eileen whispered to the baby, 'I love you. I hope you have a good life.'

And Barbara was taken away by strangers, a form of abduction sanctioned by law, to a life Eileen could never know anything about. A hole in the fabric of space opened, and the baby disappeared through it into dimensions where her mother couldn't follow.

*I hope you have a good life.* It had the feel of an epitaph – though not one for the dead. One for the living, for the vanished child.

I saw Eileen differently after she told me this story. The slapstick nature of much of her lifestyle, the raggedness around the edges of her world, the casual way she treated time and appointments and dull everyday stuff – suddenly these seemed to me elements of a life lived on a tightrope, no safety net below; a breakneck life, because she'd already been fractured and had nothing to fear from any other damage. She'd been hurt, and even if the pain had been tamped down so that it only smouldered instead of flamed, it was still there, and she could still smell it.

She'd given birth to a child, then *given that child away* – how in Christ's name did that feel to a woman? How could I ever know? Nine months and then nothing, a raw absence in the womb and no baby to feed from your nipples or hold tenderly against your shoulder. *Here, take the baby away, find it a home, I can't have it.* I couldn't make the leap into recreating these emotions. Emptiness? Sadness? Devastation? Grief? Or everything all at once, a maelstrom of feelings?

I wondered if it was akin to the emotions of a mother whose daughter had inexplicably disappeared on the way home from school one day, never to be seen again despite police searching woodlands and dragging rivers and lakes, despite all the hopes raised by the mistaken testimony of eyewitnesses claiming to have spotted the child. Never knowing where your daughter is. Never finding out. All the days of your life spent wondering. Waiting. Jumping when the phone rang, or the doorbell chimed. Or was it similar to the sorrow experienced by the mother whose child had lived a few feeble days or weeks, only to die?

The wind blew across the hills and shook the tent. Rain spattered on canvas. We drank wine and the candles spluttered and the ropes creaked, like the sound of a small sailboat anchored on a windy night. I looked at her face and waited to hear if she had anything else to add. But she didn't. She was finished with her story, and drained by the telling of it.

It would be more than thirty years before she'd say anything about her baby again.

But I knew she couldn't forget. Because even if she tried, even if she willed the memory out of existence, even if she *denied* the child had ever been born, every time she showered or bathed or changed clothes and caught sight of herself in a mirror, she'd see the scar and she'd remember, she'd always remember.

# 3

Eileen went to London in 1963 and found work with a record store on New Bond Street. I had arranged to follow her a few weeks later. The southward trek was a well-worn path. Would-be writers and artists and musicians and con men and criminals from provincial cities invariably went to London to make their mark or to fail: the provinces hadn't become fashionable yet. My parents weren't pleased; they still thought I should have finished school, and my father, in a rather old-fashioned way, considered London a place of terrible temptations for a young man. He even had a hesitant talk to me about the dangers of loose women and sexual disease, the first time he'd mentioned the subjects. He was clearly uncomfortable with them. I hadn't told either of my parents about Eileen. I had the feeling they'd bring up the age difference between us, and I didn't feel like arguing the matter.

In London, I had a variety of jobs – selling hardware in Earl's Court (without any interest in nails and nuts and screwdrivers, I was truly ill-suited for this), doing assorted clerical work, sending out dunning letters for a TV rental company to customers in arrears.

Eileen and I didn't live together. She needed a place where, if her mother had a mind to come down from Glasgow, she'd find her daughter in chaste circumstances. Doris still knew nothing of my existence. Nor did Eileen's brother Sydney; she didn't confide in him. And her father, Issy, had recently died of a heart attack, which meant that a sudden visit from a grieving Doris wasn't altogether unlikely. It astonishes me to reconstruct this fortress of subterfuge we built around our relationship. What difference would it have made if anyone had known? I realise now that what we had done was a form of elopement. A romantic flight.

Eileen rented a small flat in the nebulous area between Kilburn and Cricklewood in Northwest London. For a time I lived in an attic in what had once been a very grand house in Belsize Park but was now an intricate labyrinth of small partitioned rooms inhabited by Chinese, Indians, Pakistanis, West Indians and an Australian playwright who lived and worked in a walk-in closet. It was a riotous house, filled with babble and the perfume of exotic spices. My attic room had a leaky gas ring on the floor beside the bed. If I'd been suicidal during the night, there would have been no need to get up to gas myself. There was a sink in the corner that didn't drain very well. The nearest bathroom was down one flight of stairs, and it was invariably occupied by an irate Chinaman whom I suspected of sleeping in the bathtub. The place was squalid, of course it was, but it didn't look that way to me. Bedraggled, maybe. But mine. My very own garret.

This was a whole new world and who cared about sinks that took days to drain anyway? It was 1962 in London, a vigorous city at a vigorous time, the air zapped with electricity, a bohemian life, literary chinwagging with other wannabee writers in the pubs, drip-flecked painters who worked in lofts, late-night Chinese and Indian restaurants that made you giddy with scents of ginger and cumin and garam masala and chilies, Italian joints with candles in straw-jacketed chianti bottles, starry drunkenness on beer or cheap wine along the Finchley Road.

I liked drunkenness as a condition, the swivelling of my perceptions, the unfettered rush of thought, the laughable clumsiness of speech, the dizziness, the unexpected verbal intimacies drunken strangers share. *I'll let you in on a secret, I never told anybody, but my wife is having an affair . . . Lissename, I wanna tell you about my brother, he's a poof, a fucking poof, the family's mortified . . .*

Being drunk was like belonging to a union with no regulations, only a nominal membership fee, the price of perhaps four or five pints of beer – and no benefits beyond the easy camaraderie of booze. Drink gladdened my heart, and besides, I wasn't yet old enough to be victimised by hangovers. As for the word 'alcoholic' – it would never have entered my mind that any of the people I drank with were alcoholics. The very idea that *I* might be travelling that road – whoa, let's not be preposterous. Alkies were gutter people, devastated inhabitants of dosshouses, they blinked in the daylight like decrepit old pit ponies brought up from the bottom of the mineshaft after a score of years in the deep dank black of the earth. OK, I liked to drink, but that was it. I knew when to stop. I had control. Yes indeed. Besides, when you'd done a soul-grinding day's work trying to repossess TVs from houses in Islington or East Ham filled with Nigerians who all had the same name but none ever had the TV you were seeking, you needed relief and a working arrangement with inebriation.

Eileen drank with me, but her thirst was nowhere as intense as mine. A couple of vodka tonics, or a glass or two of wine, a sensible drinker. I have no recollection of her being drunk – a little lopsided maybe, giggling, but never out of control. In any event, she preferred exploring London to sitting in bars. She was hugely enthused by the place, and energised. Her kind of city, great and romantic and fun, far more hospitable then than it is now, an enchanting place before it was shafted by developers and cheapened by chain stores. We walked miles together, the Embankment, the Serpentine, Speaker's Corner, Regent's Park Zoo, Kew. We behaved like weekend tourists – a day at Lord's watching cricket (Eileen snoozed through the experience), a great gathering on a glorious red autumn morning in Trafalgar Square to hear a frail Bertrand Russell speak on behalf of the Campaign for Nuclear Disarmament, buying tickets to see Ella Fitzgerald at the Embassy in Kilburn. We ate in inexpensive restaurants up and down Kilburn High Road. Our favourite was the surreal Old Prague, unintentionally international, delightfully slapstick and slapdash, Italian food served on stolen British European Airways plates by waiters who spoke only Czech. Eileen might have been a small child set loose in a palace of many wonders. The constraints of Glasgow were four hundred miles to the north. Down here, she was truly free. And so was I.

For my birthday in 1964 she bought me a typewriter, the first I'd ever owned, an Olivetti manual portable with a black-red ribbon. I knew she couldn't afford it, and that she was making weekly payments on it, which made the gift all the more touching. I set aside the Big Novel and began to work on TV plays, sometimes delivering them in person to the BBC in Shepherd's Bush (as if the personal touch might help: *here, mate, see if you can get this truly amazing script to the right people*), and handing them to a uniformed commissionaire who didn't give a damn. In my memory, it is always raining in

Shepherd's Bush. The scripts never failed to come back, often without comment. I wasn't deterred. Depressed maybe, but never defeated. It was perhaps the most important lesson for any aspiring writer – beyond considerations of plot and character and style and other textbook concepts: if you can't persist, forget it.

I have no precise recollection of the moment when Eileen told me she was pregnant. It happened about the same time as I learned I'd been accepted at Sussex University. I'd never had any intention of going to university, I hadn't the necessary qualifications anyhow, but Sussex had a scheme whereby a few students could enter on the basis of an interview and an essay. I sent off for the application the way some people might do a crossword puzzle, idly, absent-mindedly. I was asked to write an essay on A J Ayer's *Language Truth & Logic,* which I did; I was surprised and pleased when Sussex offered me a place a month later.

But now a baby had entered the scheme of our lives. What were we going to do with a *baby*? The notion of fatherhood, responsibility – I was only twenty years old, I wasn't prepared, fatherhood seemed completely foreign to me, I wasn't ready to be anyone's Dad. What sort of things were expected of you? What were you supposed to know, and what could you learn and were there books to read and on and on? I skirted the edges of panic. Eileen, after an initial period of uncertainty, was calm. She began to look forward to the arrival of the child. Was this a replacement for the one she had to give away? Had she longed for this? She never mentioned Barbara during this time; maybe part of her wanted to believe that the child she carried now was her first, that Barbara belonged in another lifetime, another dimension. That child was gone, unrecoverable. Or maybe the memory of Barbara, and the mystery of her whereabouts, was too hurtful to ever consider again. Or perhaps, in her own most hidden recesses, in that place where all your most troublesome questions are left unasked, she wondered.

We both knew the baby was the end of the secrecy that surrounded our relationship. A child was something you just couldn't conceal. Sooner or later, her mother would have to know, and so would my parents. But we postponed telling them. Somehow it was never the time.

Eileen urged me to go to Sussex, but I was reluctant because of the pregnancy. She came up with a plan: I'd spend the weekdays in Brighton, while she remained in London and continued to work, and I'd return to be with her at weekends. I wasn't happy with this scheme, I didn't like the separation and I didn't like her being on her own. She argued that it would be folly to pass up the chance to go to university, and I'd regret it later.

I could arrange the finance easily enough by means of a direct grant – so money didn't enter the equation of our lives for once. I simply didn't want to leave her. What if there were complications with the baby? What if something went wrong and I couldn't be reached? What if what if . . . It was a balancing act. I couldn't leave, I couldn't stay. We discussed marriage, decided it was something we'd get round to; there was no urgency. Another postponement. We lived a life of adjournments and deferments. Tomorrow, there was always tomorrow. Why decide anything today?

By this time we'd begun living together. I couldn't take the attic existence any more; I'd foolishly allowed a very bad Scottish folk band by the name of McDougall, McNab and McKay – three accordion players, God help me – to spend a night on my floor, and they showed no inclination to leave. Weeks passed and the band members, surrounded by their instrument cases, slid into a kind of terminal drunken stupor, and the scummy sink became utterly clogged, draining at a rate of about an eighth of an inch a day. Also, the band had begun to develop a smell, and at night when they took off their socks I noticed how, even without feet in them, the socks were stiff enough to stand without help. Altogether, it was a situation more easily abandoned than resolved. I simply packed my stuff and walked out one morning and never returned.

Eileen and I rented a two-room flat in Willesden Green on a respectable leafy street whose only notoriety was that the Rolling Stones lived directly opposite us. I used to see the word MICK chalked on walls (how innocent, no spraypaint), and clutches of girls hanging around. Who or what was MICK? The Rolling Stones hadn't yet become famous. I took MICK to be a political acrostic of Irish origin, because this neighbourhood was filled with Irish immigrants.

In the late summer of 1964, I travelled by train the fifty miles from Victoria Station to Brighton, torn between thinking of babies and nappies and R H Tawney's *Religion & The Rise of Capitalism*, the first textbook I was expected to read. I remember feeling sad, listening to the click-clack rhythms of the wheels and looking out across grassy fields already past the prime of ripeness. The year was sliding towards autumn.

Brighton – magical and shabby, a grand old dame of the sea-side whose tiara is askew and ballgown stained: living on in illusion and nostalgia, clinging to her Regency heritage, the fine old squares and crescents and houses of wonderful pro-portion, the two piers – the rather sedate West (at this time of writing, alas a wreck) and the gaudy show-us-yer-knickers Palace – lacy white wood and intricate iron fretwork jutting out into the grey-brown waters of the English Channel. A resort town, different from the Scarborough where Eileen had given birth to the baby Barbara in 1955, Brighton had long been a favourite of Londoners on weekend trips, its name synonymous with dirty weekends and hotel registers signed 'Mr and Mrs J Smith'.

I moved into university accommodation in town. The university was less than a year old, and had developed a trendy liberal reputation. It was *the* hip campus, always being written about in newspapers and magazines; it became a fashionable alternative for students who might otherwise have gone to Oxford or Cambridge. Lectures were not compulsory at Sussex, and so I attended only one in my three years there. The student was left largely to his or her own devices, apart from a weekly tutorial or two. I didn't study hard, only enough to squeeze through.

I travelled to the campus, some four miles out of town, a couple of days a week. The social life of the university didn't interest me. I preferred the bars you could find in the narrow working-class backstreets of Kemp Town, away from the main tourist drags along the seafront, or the student haunts. I drank more than I studied; some days I skipped tutorials because I was beginning to develop hangovers, slight ones, little nuisances compared to the full-grown monsters they'd become later. (But what was I doing drinking like this? I was supposed to be working towards a degree, a piece of paper that would enrich my life and Eileen's and our baby's, something that would help us get wherever we were going. She believed in me. What was I trying to do – ruin it all? I'd make resolutions to quit or cut down. I lived inside interconnecting boxes of resolutions. Don't drink. Work harder. Go to more lectures. Study more.)

I liked Brighton, but I was missing Eileen. The weekend trips back to London were pleasant, but not enough. Some nights, I wondered about her, and how she passed time alone.

I'd imagine her rising, still slim yet; I'd picture her travelling by tube to work, I'd see her serving customers – conscientious, helpful, patient, she was always these things; I'd imagine her returning to the small flat in Willesden Green at about seven o'clock in the evening and how tired she was of being on her feet all day, I'd see her kick off her shoes, make herself coffee, light a cigarette, flick the pages of a book or magazine, watch a little TV, listen to music. I'd think of her running the palm of her hand across her stomach, feeling the scar, remembering, not remembering. I'd imagine her as she slept, the foetus taking shape inside her, the small hands, fingers forming, the blind eyes, this unborn baby fumbling towards consciousness and light, this stranger. She never complained about being alone; she was determined that I finish university.

Pregnancy was changing her in more ways than the physical; as she developed a bond with the child she was becoming quieter, even sedate. At weekends she preferred to stay at home. No more long walks through London, no more flippant tube rides to unknown destinations whose names whimsically took our fancy – Cockfosters, Clapham, Crawley. She was moving into domesticity, into motherhood. A different Eileen – she was evolving. She had our child in her womb; the centre of her universe had altered.

Even as she grew in size, she continued to work. On Christmas Eve, 1964, she finished her last day on the job, and on 28 December she went into hospital where, the following morning, she gave birth to a boy we named Iain.

And now it was time, finally, to tell our parents.

My mother and father took the news with reasonable calm, and questions like *Why didn't you tell us? Didn't you think we might have helped out?* But we were worried less about telling my parents than we were about relaying the news to Doris –

who hadn't recovered from the death of her husband – her
life-partner was gone, her entire support system collapsed.
Life without him was a dreary prospect and she was sunk in
despondency, as if she were merely marking time until her
own death. Eileen wrote or telephoned – I don't remember
which now – to tell her about Iain.

Shocked, Doris announced that she was coming down to
England as soon as she could make the necessary arrangements, whatever they were. By this time, we'd moved to
Brighton and had a flat just beyond the railway station, in an
area called Seven Dials. Eileen gently broached the subject of
her mother living with us for a time, at least until she knew
what she was going to do with her life. I had no objections. I'd
met Doris a few years ago in Cuthbertson's, when she'd
dropped in to the shop to see Eileen, but I couldn't have said
that I *knew* her. We'd nodded at one another, a quick exchange
of names. There was a spare room in the flat and Doris could
use it, if she wanted to stay.

And so Doris duly arrived, with suitcases. She was a small
silver-haired woman with thick-lensed glasses that made her
eyes big, and a certain air of drama about her. She studied me
for a time – avoiding the subject of Iain. She said nothing, but
her look was mildly accusing: *So you're the one? You're the
father? A boy like you? A student, penniless?*

And then she turned to Eileen and took a very deep breath
and her hands trembled as she said, 'Give me a minute before
I see this baby.' She appeared to undergo some kind of internal struggle, and I wondered if she was remembering another
baby years before Iain, if Scarborough had crossed her mind.
If she was thinking about the time when she and her late husband had been together with Eileen in that town by the North
Sea. If she was remembering how she'd done everything in her
power to protect her young daughter's future.

She composed herself after a moment and said she was ready now to see the baby. Eileen brought Iain to her. Doris took the child in her arms. 'He's got grey eyes,' she whispered. *'He's got his grandfather's eyes.'*

And I understood: Iain was a life in return for a death. Iain was a form of compensation for the late Issy, a substitute of sorts. In grief we look for the spaces left by our losses to be filled; we seek out similarities, coincidences, omens, signs. We want life to have meaningful alignments, because otherwise the deaths of our loved ones are random cruelties in a cruelly random universe.

Doris held the baby to her body. From that moment on, everything was accepted and acceptable – me, the baby, Eileen and I as partners. I wasn't the penniless student, the goyim boy, suddenly I was an aspiring writer with ambition, I was a man going places in life. And the baby – no child could have been more fussed-over, adored, than Iain.

Doris took control of running the household. She separated the meat from the dairy dishes, in kosher fashion. Pots and pans were similarly segregated.

After a time, I felt relaxed enough around her to make the kind of little jokes that are grounded in familiarity. She smoked cigarettes constantly, and always had one dangling from her lip when she cooked, and I'd watch the ash grow long as she forgot about the fact she was smoking and I'd ask, *Didn't we have cigarette-ash soup last night, Doris?* Or I'd bring a piece of steak home and tell her I'd bought it at the kosher butcher, and she wasn't sure if she could believe me or not, and consequently the steak was deemed to be of uncertain provenance and was discarded (it didn't matter that we were poor, of course). Or I'd tell her I'd accidentally spilled milk in the chicken she had in the refrigerator and I'd tried to wipe it off with a paper towel. She was never sure if I was being truthful at these times; she'd look at me through those enormous magnified eyes and her uncertainty would yield to head-shaking laughter. She had a smoker's hoarse hack of a chuckle, and she always bent over during it. She rarely laughed briefly, it was usually a prolonged business, as if she were truly delighted by mirth; maybe she'd imagined, after the death of Issy, that it was something she'd never feel again.

Once or twice I had the overwhelming need to grill a piece of forbidden bacon for a sandwich. Consequently, I found myself smuggling the verboten substance into the house as if it were heroin, and concealing it, then waiting until Doris had gone upstairs to sleep before I slapped the strips on the grill and cooked them. Once, halfway through this enterprise, I heard her descend. Creak creak on the stairs. Oh God, the bacon was sizzling and curling on the grill, and had reached that delightful stage when its fumes fill the room, and I knew, I just *knew* there could be no escape from Doris's annoyance, her wrath even, what was I doing cooking swine flesh in her kosher kitchen? What contamination was this? What sacrilege? I opened the window and grabbed the bacon strips from the grill and shoved them under the sink and waved my arms frantically to dispel the aroma; but bacon doesn't go away in a twinkling.

Doris stepped inside the kitchen, walked to the sink, filled a glass of water and said, 'Woke up feeling thirsty.'

I waited. She looked at me over the rim of her glass. She's going to mention the smell, I thought. I had no lie prepared. What could I have dreamed up anyway? *Doris, you wouldn't believe it, I confronted a burglar who just happened to be taking a break in his work to enjoy a bacon sandwich?*

She walked to the kitchen doorway, paused, looked back at me.

'Isn't it a wee bit on the *cold* side to have the windows open?' she asked.

And then she went back up to her room.

She knew. I knew she knew. She knew I knew she knew. From that time on, there was a bond between us, a tiny conspiracy of sorts. If an argument arose, if Eileen and I disagreed over something, Doris invariably took my side. When Eileen and I moved from Brighton to London she came with us, and she stayed for a time before she decided she was homesick. I was a little sorry to see her go back to Glasgow in the end.

In 1977, she died as her husband had done, suddenly.

# 4

THIS is what Stephen says on that summer day in 1997 in Ireland after he reaches the top of the stairs: 'She has malignant tumours in both lungs. They're inoperable.'

Inoperable is a club to the side of my brain. It's a word physicians use when they're obliged to admit their own uselessness. They've reached the borderline of their knowledge and they don't know what lies in the territory beyond. One day, an intrepid explorer will hack into that jungle, but so far there has been no authentic Columbus of Cancer.

I react by saying what you usually say in those situations where language is inapplicable, and words are as substantial as bubblegum balloons. 'No, it's a mistake. Has to be.'

'It doesn't sound like it. The X-rays—'

'X-rays can be misinterpreted. How did she take the news?'

'I didn't talk to her,' Stephen says. 'Nancy told me.'

Nancy Frick, Eileen's best friend and co-worker, a solid presence in Eileen's life. I imagine Eileen, crushed by this damning verdict, shocked and hysterical, asking Nancy to break the news to family and friends.

Stephen sits down on the steps that lead to the door of my study. I sit beside him and we say nothing for a time. I want to do something decisive, seize the situation by the scruff of the neck, dredge something up from the depths of myself that will ease Stephen: but I'm empty, and I'm also in a state of shocked disbelief. I'd like to turn the clock back just a couple of minutes to that point in time before he made the phone call, where everything was sane and normal and the early evening sky blue and wonderful, but now the world is upside down.

Stephen says, 'What are we going to do.'

It isn't really a question. He has another week of his vacation left to him here – but I already know he isn't going to stay that length of time. I know he's thinking of flying back home to Phoenix to be with his mother. I need to tell Rebecca this news of Eileen, but it hasn't penetrated yet to the point where it's absolute fact in my head. There's still some kind of glaze between myself and reality. And telling Rebecca isn't going to be easy, because she's always had respect and affection for Eileen. Christ, just saying it *aloud* isn't going to be easy.

My son's expression is bleak. He has problems other than his mother – he's separated from his wife and kids and he's in Ireland because he has the idea he might have peace and space here to work things out in his mind, come to some solution. Now his marital situation, already fragile, is overshadowed by Eileen's diagnosis. I wonder how he'll handle all this.

I think of the other sons Eileen and I have, Iain in Phoenix, Keiron in Seattle: have they had the news of their mother yet? Suddenly I wish the boys and I were together, that we weren't scattered across the planet. I want the comfort of blood-ties. How long has it been since we were all together, Eileen included, anyhow? Stephen's wedding is the last occasion I can recall, and that was seven years before, when he was twenty. It's a long time. Too long. But then our family life has been fractured for a while, particles spinning off in different directions.

For a time we sit on the steps motionless. He talks about changing his ticket, wonders if he can catch a flight back the next day. He says he'll call the airline: do I mind if he cuts his holiday short? Do I *mind*? What else can he do in the circumstances? I hug him: there's a sense of impending loss. If he goes tomorrow the house will feel diminished for a time – but beyond that loss lies another potential one I don't even want to entertain, the idea of Eileen and cancer, of her succumbing to it. How little I know about cancer: it's what happens in the next house, the next street. It's what strikes down distant aunts, cousins you barely know. When it comes to perch on your own roof, you have to accommodate its strange force because you can't demand that it leave. It's the deadly gate-crasher that stays until the party is well and truly done. It takes possession of lives.

Stephen goes downstairs to get the phone number of the airline. Sun comes through the skylights above the staircase. The sky should be grey, the evening rainy and miserable; bad news weather. But the light is lovely and persistent, and the day refuses to die.

I tell Rebecca when we're alone. The news upsets her as I knew it would. She asks how Stephen is taking it. I tell her he's arranging to fly back to the United States the next day, if he can get a booking. She says she must speak to him alone before he goes. Rebecca has had serious tragedy in her life, the loss of twin daughters who lived only days. I know a part of her grieves still for these babies, and although the pain has subsided somewhat over the years it will never leave her entirely. Consequently, she's quick to empathise with the sick, quick to help and understand. I think of my ex-wife alone with her diagnosis; I try to imagine my present wife alone at the time of her own past tragedy. There's a place of dread in every tragedy or illness when the well-wishers and the comforters go home, or when those around the sickbed must leave, or spouses need sleep or they have to go out to work, and you're left in solitude: in all the world it's just you and your condition – be it disease, bereavement, whatever the pain. There's the inevitable moment when you carry it alone, and you must feel very small and your life an impossible one, but you know you have to find the will from somewhere to go on. The miracle that astonishes me is that people *do* find it in the most arctic conditions of the human heart. Courage, strength, a deep inner tributary of bravery, call it by any of those names: somehow we endure. Somehow we persist.

I suggest to Rebecca that perhaps Eileen's condition isn't as bad as we imagine, that we won't know for sure until I've talked to her on the telephone, or Stephen has had a chance to see her. Rebecca reacts in a subdued way to these remarks. Inoperable is the word that straitjackets her. She says specialists use that word when there's usually only one outcome, and it's not good, and she has a look of dismay. I'm balancing on the high wire of maybes . . . maybe this, maybe that, but there's no real strength in the rope. Rebecca's feelings for Eileen's plight are apparent in her manner, that sorrow in her eyes, the way she works the tips of her thumbs together in a characteristic gesture of worry, and I suddenly think how fortunate my life has been that I have known and married two very different but exceptional women. I have a right to my optimism, if that's what it is.

We go in search of Stephen. He's made his travel arrangements. He'll fly out of Shannon the next day. Rebecca tells him how sorry she is and holds him, but I know she has more she wants to say, and she'll wait for a moment of privacy.

As light fades, I walk with Stephen in the pine woods around our house. The pathway is quiet, the woods secretive, the air scented. Everywhere there are reminders of life. In birdsong, leaf, shrub, the tremble of a branch disturbed by a crow's landing. I hear myself ramble on in a voice that's not really my own – we need to get a second opinion, I read just recently how they're making great strides in chemotherapy these days, cancer's not the death sentence it used to be – but I run out of speech. I'm doing exactly what I don't want to, I'm doling out useless anodynes. I can't help myself. Am I really so relentlessly upbeat? Is this how some people see me? Stephen does me the kindness of nodding in mute agreement to each of my offerings; or maybe he simply wants to grasp one of these little capsules of hope I'm passing in front of him.

We come to a place where pathways intersect and we sit on an old log. Wild strawberries grow in rich clusters. I pick a few, eat them; they detonate sweetly in the mouth. Stephen plucks some, declares them delicious. For a time neither of us can stop, we go at the tiny berries with gusto, our fingertips turning blood-red. He won't be here this time tomorrow, I think. The strawberries will still be clustered on the branches, but we won't be here together to eat them like this. This strikes me as unbearably sad – it's distance again, it's time and space. It's absence. It's knowing he's flying back to see his mother. To see for himself how sick she is.

'You don't want to eat too many of these,' he says, his voice serious and responsible. 'Blood sugar levels. Remember?'

I still have to force myself to keep diabetes in mind – but compared to cancer it seems more an inconvenience than an ailment with potentially serious consequences. I have to watch my intake of sugar and swallow one gliclazide tab a day and in all likelihood I'll live a long enough life; what can Eileen ingest that will carry the same promise? What kind of pill do you swallow when it comes to haywire cells in the lung? Mutating outrages, tumours, what kind of defence is there against them?

'Screw blood sugar levels,' I say. 'These are too good.'

We eat some more. We're like truant schoolboys, wary of discovery. It's a great moment, two red-lipped gluttons in the forest at twilight. It's something to be remembered later with pleasure. For a short while it's possible to set aside the way this day has turned out and avoid what lies ahead. We smoke cigarettes, walk a little further along the path in silence and then, because night is falling, we turn back.

The house is lit. Inside, Rebecca and Stephen drink a little wine and talk together while I wander without direction through various rooms. I think of calling Eileen, but if she doesn't want to talk to anyone yet then I must respect that. I go upstairs to my office. Darkness is spreading across the fields. The night is starry. Three days from now it will be 21 June, the longest day of the year. Midsummer Night. I sit at the keyboard, look absently at the arrangement of letters in front of me. The house is unusually silent. What time is it in Arizona? Again I think of telephoning. No, let it be.

I wonder what Stephen and Rebecca are saying to each other and I think about the history between them, the textbook nature of it – of how, when Stephen came to live with Rebecca and me, shortly after my divorce from Eileen, he ran away from home with some of his friends and ended up all the way across the country in Florida; or the time when he was living with us and got involved in a joy-riding incident and a high-speed chase with the Arizona State Police on the day he'd promised to be best man at my wedding to Rebecca. There are wounds in all this, old sores that haven't healed, residual resentments. Rebecca has forgiven – up to a point. I know she likes Stephen because he's easy to like, but whether she can trust him is another matter; whether *he* can ever love and appreciate *her* is another matter still. They have forged a pleasant working truce over the years, which I suspect is for my sake; all I want is for each to see what *I* see in them – caring, generous human beings. Stephen happens to have taken a couple of wrong turnings. So what? Who hasn't?

They are two of the people I love most in this world.

There's still the taste of strawberries in my mouth. I hear Stephen come up the stairs. Rebecca is with him. She's been crying, I can tell. Stephen looks a little pale, but he's smiling. He has a good smile. Big and friendly. Suddenly the mood is light for no reason – release, maybe. A few minutes out of reality. The air might be filled with down or dandelion filaments. This is a world where nobody is sick. Everybody is healthy forever. Stephen records a silly message in a thick Scottish accent on my computer, designed to play every time I switch on or off. *What are ye gonna do?* This question is destined to become a kind of family in-joke, something that gets repeated until it grows wearisome. But it's a good question. All-purpose. Applicable to every situation. Smart kid sometimes, Stephen.

I drive him next morning to Shannon, fifty miles. He's subdued. I detect a touch of apprehension in him, more than the usual pre-flight anxieties. He's thinking of his mother, what he's going to find when he gets to his destination. I want to ask what it was he and Rebecca discussed the previous evening, but I don't like to intrude. If he's going to bring it up, he will. An Irish rain is falling; it's the kind they call 'soft' around here. Quiet, sweeping the fields, everything is grey and drab. Damp sheep, huddled cows, farmers working glistening tractors in black fields that suck on fat tires, an evil whiff of pig slurry deteriorating on the air.

Stephen tells me he had a 'heavy' conversation with Rebecca.

Heavy? I ask what this means.

He seems reluctant to say any more; whatever he's shared with Rebecca is between him and her. He will only tell me this much – that she's explained to him what she holds to be incontrovertibly true: no matter what happens to Eileen, she will *always* be with Stephen. Always. After life, she will be there in some form. This is Rebecca's firm conviction: life goes on after physical annihilation. Whether as some kind of consciousness, some form of ethereal echo, life goes on. And so it will be with Eileen. No matter what. Rebecca subscribes to no religious views. She isn't a member of any church. She has a serious aversion to organised religion. But this is her one constant spiritual belief: death is not an end. And whenever she speaks about this, there's absolutely no question about how deeply she feels it to be true. It's not a tenet I share easily; but I wouldn't argue the point with her.

And now I look into the rainy morning and I think why not give credence to the survival of consciousness after death? What is there to lose anyhow? It's Pascal's old wager.

Stephen says, 'I enjoyed talking with her. She opened up. She told me about the two daughters that died.'

I say I'm glad. And I am. The idea of them communicating pleases me. I wish the subject matter had been different, that's all. I wish they'd had something light-hearted to confer about, another kind of sharing. Was Rebecca quietly trying to prepare Stephen for the worst? I imagine she came at it gently, circuitously, if that's what she was doing. More likely she just wants to share her belief with him, and some of her past experience of bad times. This is it, Stephen. This is where I stand. I want you to know.

Now rain falls harder the closer we get to Shannon. This is the time I hate, the farewell, I'm never any good at it – and in these circumstances I'm less than good. I'm melting down.

'You'll phone as soon as you see your mother,' I say.

'I promise.'

'You won't forget.'

Stephen reassures me. He won't forget. He'll call as soon as he gets the chance. We walk in the direction of the departures gate. When he shows his passport and goes through that door with the sign Passengers Only then he's lost to me, and I can't follow, I can't add anything to what's already been said, no afterthoughts, no further talk. He'll step past the uniformed guard and disappear up the escalator and he'll turn once and wave, and that will be it.

I hug him for a long time. And then he goes.

I trudge outside through the rain to my car and I drive away from Shannon without looking back. All you see are planes rising into the clouds, carrying people away. People you wish didn't have to leave. Never look back.

# 5

4 July 1997, Independence Day. I fly out of Dublin to Phoenix, Arizona, from the cool and tolerable to the hot and unbearable; exchanging the convivial city alongside the murky Liffey for the vast shapeless mass of Phoenix which, with its crowded satellite towns, always reminds me of a big brown pod split open by the fierce heat and its fat seeds spilled. Seven years have passed since I left the United States, and I'm flying back into uncertainty, a man without a compass. I look at Dublin recede, and then the green island-nation is sucked behind clouds and we are climbing out across the Atlantic.

I immediately have one of those nicotine attacks hooked smokers experience when they're trapped in an airborne cylinder for some ten hours. Cigarettes, cigarettes: how many years of her life has Eileen spent smoking? She quit – when – seven years ago? Eight? I saw her at Stephen's wedding but I can't remember if she was smoking that day. We've talked by telephone, letter, fax and e-mail, but why can't I recall our last face-to-face meeting? My memory won't yield an answer. I'm blocking recollections of that wedding day; maybe it's because I don't want to compare how she last looked to the image I have of how she might look now.

I watch the in-flight attendants go up and down the aisles, and the notion of having a drink drifts through my head: I haven't had alcohol in years. The notion fizzles quickly. We had a falling-out, booze and I, after a few miserable wrecked truces.

At thirty-five thousand feet I tear open a bag of peanuts upside down and they spill to the floor. A friendly passenger, an American going home, laughs at my clumsiness and helps me gather them up, and I realise I've forgotten the easygoing nature of certain Americans, the compulsive openness that makes them want to go straight to first names – hey, I'm Clay – and before long you're looking at photographs of MaryJo and little Brad and Bobbie back in Macon, Georgia, and the scent of a remembered barbecue blows through your mind.

I need this kind of company for the moment. I need the reassurance of MaryJo and Clay and the kids and hickory or mesquite burning, an attachment to the ordinary. Because I don't really know where I'm going, and what I'll find when I get there. I think of Eileen sliding down a very dark slope of illness. And I am halfway out across the Atlantic, afraid for her, afraid for the sons we have had together. The sons who love her, the sons I love.

Change planes at Atlanta, an airport of fluorescent enormity. Living for seven years on the edge of a tiny Irish village, I've grown unaccustomed to the drift of people in large numbers, the immense commerce of conveying them from place to place; where I live, our idea of mass transport is the bus that carries fifty people to bingo sessions in the village hall on

Thursday nights. Like a backwater rube, I wander in a disoriented fashion under the great banks of arrivals and departures consoles. Hundreds of mainline flights, and commuter connections on airlines I've never heard of.

Phoenix, I am looking for Phoenix, and for some time can't find it; a kind of odd little panic comes over me. Reno, Las Vegas, Albuquerque, Salt Lake City, Seattle. Everything but the place I'm looking for. Where's Phoenix? Has the flight been cancelled? Has the city been written out of the schedules entirely? Or meltdown in the fierce heat? I don't want to go to Phoenix anyway, I realise. Be honest. You wish you didn't have a reason to come to the United States (especially a reason like the one that brings you here now). But you do. You wish you were home with Rebecca. But you're not. How very far away she seems. Dreamlike. My sense of time has been deconstructed. I'd taken melatonin on the flight but hadn't slept – now I'm groggy, spacey, which might explain the hallucinogenic feel of the terminal building and the great flux of seemingly expressionless people.

Phoenix, *Phoenix*: finally I locate it on the board, memorise the gate number, forget it immediately, re-check it, then the need to smoke assaults me. I discover the Smoking Lounge (smokers have the instincts of truffle hunters), a small primitive room that reeks like a million ashtrays. It has no amenities, no comforts. This is where you are sent if you have the Habit. It's the airport version of the leper colony. I go inside, light up, look around. The other addicts have the intensity of people about to face a firing squad: the cigarette each one smokes is the last before he or she is taken out and shot.

Every so often a nonsmoker passes the window of the Lounge and looks in as if he were gazing into a cage at a zoo. Hundreds of years from now, in a perfect smoke-free world, this Lounge will be preserved as a museum piece. *Twentieth-*

*Century Addictions: The Smoking Room*. It will be filled with androids holding holographs of cigarettes. Tour parties will peer through the window and listen to a guide recite the history of tobacco abuse.

Suddenly I resent myself and the way I'm impaled on a lethal addiction. But it's more than self-resentment, more than my preoccupation with a bad habit. It's Eileen. The association between her and tobacco has been playing in my mind for hours now. I wonder how she is, what she's thinking, feeling. We were once so close. I try to imagine her horror. I can't get to that level.

I remember Rebecca telling me: *You must go to Arizona. Your sons need you. Eileen needs you. Especially now.* I admire my wife's benevolent spirit.

Another show of unselfishness comes back to me from that terrible time when my marriage with Eileen had come as unglued as a book with a worm-eaten binding, and I'd met Rebecca and found myself impossibly divided between two lives: a marriage that had flopped and wilted, and the possibility of a more fulfilling future with another woman. It wasn't a situation conducive to general merriment; my obvious unhappiness made Eileen genuinely miserable. And Rebecca found herself on an emotional expressway, looking for the nearest exit ramp; she was determined she wouldn't become that creature of vilification, the 'other woman'.

Eileen appeared unexpectedly one day at the door of Rebecca's apartment when Rebecca was alone. With a stunning generosity of heart I knew caused her deep pain, she said she felt that I would only be happy if I could be with Rebecca. So – and this is a sacrifice only those who love unselfishly understand – she was prepared to step aside and let us get on with our lives together.

I remember Eileen's face later that day, the pale hurt look, the shocked appearance in the brown eyes, as if she couldn't believe what she'd said, or the step she'd taken. I remember what she said to me after she'd spoken with Rebecca: *I just gave you away.* She'd stepped inside her car and I made a move to call out to her, perhaps to detain her, say something, anything, repair the damages, make everything well again, God knows what, but she'd already gone out of the parking lot and, in a sense, out of my life.

There was suffering, of course, and there was anguish, and not just for Eileen. After the divorce, though, the pain didn't explode into flames of acrimony, or the incendiary bitterness that kills feeling; divorcees often allow old loves to sink into the negativity of spite and rage, which cancels out all the good years and the fun times and the love that existed in the first place. That early love changes; it undergoes a chemical alteration. It isn't what it was. But that doesn't mean it has ceased to exist entirely. Only its form is different. Not all divorces end in the blood-filled offices of expensive lawyers where the tables are strewn with stained documents attesting to disputed ownership of this meaningless object or that, and the air smells of burnt flesh and the cordite of spite, and only those vultures of misery, the attorneys, profit from bitterness.

Now I walk out of the Smoking Lounge down air-conditioned corridors towards the departures gate. I love Eileen in my way. We have three sons. Rebecca knows what I shared with my first wife and it doesn't threaten her. And now I am going to the only destination for me. Anywhere else is out of the question. I have to be going this way. And it's not something you can do just by picking up a phone and asking, Say, kids, how's your mother? And there are no excuses for refuge – I can't make it over there to be with you, very busy, maybe later. It's a time for truth.

My head's crowded with the spectres of other people's feelings. What are the boys going through? Iain, the oldest, serious and studious, a private young man who finds it hard to be demonstrative. Keiron, the youngest, who makes conversations with strangers and strikes up friendships out of nothing and who lives only to play his music. And Stephen, middle son – is it only three weeks since I put him on a plane at Shannon? We've communicated daily by phone or e-mail. He's always sounded flat on the phone, and pessimistic.

I even talked with Eileen a couple of days after her original diagnosis in June. She tried to tell me what the horror of it was like, how she experienced twenty-four hours of numbness in a place she described as 'strange and silent'. She'd thought she'd be told she had pneumonia or maybe TB at the very worst, but *lung cancer* – that was the last thing she expected.

That conversation is ten days old. Since then her situation has become worse – she's undergone emergency surgery to have a tumour lasered from her windpipe. The tumour had grown out of one lung and clogged her air passage to the extent she almost died of suffocation on a hot Phoenix street just a few days ago and was rushed to the ER. I think of her choking and going into panic and light fading from her vision and paramedics with oxygen cylinders and an ambulance racing to a hospital.

I think of the kids. Of their sadness. Fear of loss. The sharp anxiety of the unknown. I need them as much as they need me at this time, because the same sadness unites us and the same fear stalks us. And so I have come six thousand miles because I have no idea of the time left to my former wife, or if there's a bright prognosis to come – or whether the cancer has spread and the engine of the disease is already running faster and louder.

The jet rattles down the runway at Sky Harbor Airport in Phoenix and slows to a halt.

*

During the descent, I've noticed black rectangles beyond the orange illuminated runways. Wasteland, scrub, shadows that suggest mysteries, secrets. Across the world, in northern England, in a small Yorkshire town I've never visited nor even heard of, something secret is moving out of darkness towards the light.

And neither Eileen, nor me, nor our sons, know anything about it. We can't know that it is soon to take form and emerge from the buried past and, like a heatwave firing the dead heart of winter, change the weather of our lives.

# 6

IAIN and Stephen are at the airport to meet me. They look emotionally uncertain, pleased and anxious at the same time: they're in a tough place. It's often hard to see them as young men, no longer little kids. Time and circumstance, like a couple of evil spirits, steal children away from parents. Looking at them, I sometimes experience a number of quirky little jump-cuts backward – nappies, soft toys, a sparse number of candles on birthday cakes, small red faces bright in the snowfall along the shore of Lake Ontario where we lived when we first came to America: childhoods exploding in miniature fragments of memory.

I haven't seen Iain for about two years. With his short brown hair and glasses, he projects bookishness: he's more than thirty years old, which strikes me as a preposterous trick of time, and he's a student in pursuit of a medical degree – where the hell did those years go? Our lives don't simply pass. They *evaporate*. Iain likes to dress as well as he can. He has a sense of style, but it's seriously restricted by his budget. He enjoys finding a cast-off designer jacket in a thrift shop: it's treasure to him. Stephen, thick hair and brown eyes, has a more potent physical presence than his older brother. He acted in junior theatre when he was a teenager and some of the actor's projection, and ability, is still present. He doesn't give a damn about clothes most of the time. He dresses for comfort and climate. Faded jeans, T-shirt. He smiles when he hugs me – his hug is fierce – and takes my bag out of my hand. Iain holds me too. I wonder what real expectations they have of me. Support, yes. Love and friendship. Beyond those, what can I give? I can't give them their mother back as she was before.

I'm hesitant to ask the boys about Eileen immediately. Let this moment where we embrace last without interruptions. I feel depleted by my trawl through time zones, rendered powerless in some way, but the presence of the boys energises me. Only Keiron is missing. He's due to fly in from Seattle a couple of hours from now. A reunion, father and three sons: Jesus, if only we'd come together in better circumstances than these. If only the reunion had been prompted by something uplifting.

Outside the terminal, a July night in Phoenix, and the blast of heat buckles me. How hot and angry summer in Maricopa County can be, even after sunset. And the days, oh God, the blue searing sunny days will be worse. The boys laugh at my sudden discomfort. I take off my black linen jacket, damp and crumpled from travel.

'Welcome back to hell,' Iain says. It's an Iain kind of thing to say. His humour leans to the black side. This time, though, he's not just referring to the weather. I know that, and so does he.

Inside the parking garage, where the air is even more crushing, I can't postpone it any longer. I ask about their mother.

Stephen hesitates before he says, 'She's in intensive care

right now. The doctor thinks the laser surgery's been a success : . .'

Laser surgery has helped her to breathe, but beyond that nobody knows anything for sure. How long she'll live. The quality of that life. If radiation will help. If chemotherapy lies in the future. If there is a future. These are imponderables. Right now, all I want to do is go to the hospital and see her. I also want to smoke.

Iain, a trained respiratory therapist, shakes his head as I light the cigarette. He doesn't have to speak, it's all in the gesture – how can you do that to yourself, Dad? Look at mother's condition. How can you commit suicide? *I've probed inside people's chests and seen what tobacco does to lungs.* He has a way of shaking his head and gazing at the ground when he knows what he wants to say but doesn't want to say it openly. He doesn't want to scold me. Stephen decides to smoke too.

Now the three of us are split into two factions: Iain stands firm on the side of good sense, Stephen and I are aligned with the forces of self-destruction. It's inscribed on Iain's face. Dumb thing to do, guys. And so it is. Stephen has excuses ready: this is a time of high stress, I can't quit yet, later. I go along with these willingly. They are the same excuses I make for myself.

Stephen and I ride in his pickup, Iain follows behind in his own vehicle, which is strictly No Smoking and fastidiously kept, in contrast to Stephen's, where the seats and floor are scattered with papers and fast-food wrappers and clothing and kiddie things. Still separated from his wife and children, he's been living something of a nomadic existence – now at his own home with his kids, then in the spare room of someone else's house, back and forth. I wonder at the turmoil in him, the combined effect of a sick mother and a withering marriage.

I compare Stephen's history with mine: it's unavoidable.

He has three sons and is separated from his wife: I have three sons and I also separated from my wife. It's difficult to steer myself away from a moment of self-accusation: if I hadn't divorced Eileen, if I'd stayed with her and tried to shore up the marriage for the sake of the children, would Stephen's life be different now? Would Iain's? And Keiron's too? It's an easy commonplace to say that dying marriages can't be saved, and that any effort to keep them alive on an artificial support system is a whole lot worse for the children than divorce. I'm not as rabidly convinced of this as I once was. As I grow older, ideas and opinions once so persuasive have developed cracks and flaws. Is the getting of wisdom the getting of ignorance? Does senility provide the ultimate insight? What the hell – these are just more imponderables, more flotsam floating in my jet-lagged skull.

I roll down my window and look at the freeway, which has grown since I was last here. Overpasses, complicated intersections, downtown construction going on. I don't know this city. I never did. And yet it is where I brought Eileen and our sons in 1976.

I look at Stephen in the dim interior of the vehicle. He seems sad under the intermittent lights along the edge of the expressway.

'She deserves better than this,' he says.

'I know she does.'

'Nobody deserves this, Dad.'

Nobody. What did Eileen ever do to anyone? She'd given over most of her adult life trying to help others. But there's no justice. Life's a game of chance. The little steel ball clicks on the wheel and it stops where it stops, and you don't have the power to change it.

'Maybe she'll get well,' Stephen says. 'You hear about remission . . .'

Remission, this is a stock word of hope, and we'll hear it again in the days ahead. We'll hear stories of people miraculously restored to life after physicians have consigned them to the slagheap of death. Old men raddled with cancer who have outlived all the predictions of doom by thirty years. People with brain tumours who are magicked into spontaneous remission. Not a trace of cancer anywhere, X-rays clear as a bell. We'll hear these stories many times. They sometimes have the feel of urban myths. Somebody who knows somebody who knows somebody who's still alive fifty years after a cancer diagnosis – only you can never quite get to the source of the story.

I flick my cigarette out the window and it sparks away into the night and I make a strict mental note like the slash of a steel-nibbed pen on paper: *Give up this fucking habit*.

Stephen glances at me and just for a moment I have the weird feeling he's about to regress to childhood and ask me that killer question no parent can ever answer. 'Why do things have to die, Daddy?'

Family pets, schoolfriends, aunts and uncles, grandparents. Why indeed, Stephen. It's in the cycle of things. Death in life. The opening of a bright flower is always followed by its closing.

But why, Daddy?

I don't know why. Nobody does.

And then we park in the hospital lot alongside Iain's pickup. He's standing outside, waiting.

'Follow me,' he says. 'I know my way round this place.' His tone of voice suggests he wishes he'd never seen the inside of this particular hospital in his life. But there's a confidence in his step suddenly, there's none of that slightly defensive, slightly shy, slouch in his walk now. He knows hospitals. He's worked in them on and off for years. He knows the score, how to talk with nurses and orderlies, he knows what doctors expect.

We walk towards the building. My energies are dipping again suddenly. I want to get inside the air-conditioned tower but I can't move fast, the heat is a brute force pressed against anything that tries to pass through it. We make it indoors. Inside is a pastel wall hung with framed photographs of former chiefs of medical staff – how self-righteous they seem in these portraits, how sure of themselves and their powers, like good solid burghers; I feel a quirky little irritation at the sight of them and I wonder, unfairly, how many patients they failed to save – and then we enter the waiting room that is reserved for families of intensive-care patients.

A soft-drink machine, a scattering of magazines, coffee tables, a bulletin board with messages and phone numbers – *Mark please call me, Sandy. For Jack Phillips, I've gone home will return at breakfast, Andrea.* The network of messages and information, the scrawls of worried people. It's the system here. It suggests a waiting room for those whose loved ones have gone off to do battle in yet another pointless distant war, and this is the place where news seeps through. *George M, Missing in Action. Pete T, Killed by Enemy Fire.*

Iain makes a phone call to the night nurse in the IC unit. He puts the handset down and says, 'It's OK. We can go up.'

I'm anxious to see Eileen. I'm also filled with the dread that I've been carrying like rosary beads since I left Dublin. We step inside the elevator. Iain looks at the floor and sighs. Stephen places a hand on my shoulder and squeezes.

Iain says, 'I still can't believe you're here, Dad.'

Nor can I. I'm pleased to see he's pleased.

# 7

SHE lies on a bed surrounded by gadgetry, high-tech boxes, wires; she's attached to an IV drip and an oxygen machine is connected to her nasal passages by transparent plastic tubes. She's opiated, eyes shut. Her hands are lightly clasped outside the bed cover, and her colour is yellowish, like a mild jaundice. Her hair, formerly auburn-red and shiny, looks dull, and there are a few strands of grey here and there – but not many. I lean over her and press my face very lightly into her scalp, careful of the wires and tubes that surround her. Her hair smells faintly of sweat. I whisper her name and touch the back of her hand, aware of both boys standing by the bed.

I'm conscious, more than anything else, of how shrunken she seems, as if she's lost two dress sizes, dwindled by an inch or two. She was never more than five foot one at any time, now she appears even less than that. But she's just come through an operation and God knows how long the cancer has been eating at her. I say her name again, thinking: she doesn't belong in this damned place.

I've never seen her look this unhealthy before. I've seen her
with colds and flus, and I've seen her go through the occasional bouts of nausea attendant on pregnancy. I've seen her
once with a dislocated collarbone and in intense pain through
which she was able to smile nevertheless, because she's strong,
she's always had fortitude. But I've never seen her look like
this. A sick stranger.

Iain says, 'Mom. It's Dad.' There's a hopeful little plea in
his voice. He wants this information to surprise her into alert-
ness, and the return of her old self.

She doesn't respond. I speak her name a few more times.
Cancer, this monstrous claw – it rips out not only the fibre of
the body, but the threads of dignity too. She's aged. The disease has drawn knife-lines in her face. The flesh under her jaw
is slack. Her bridgework, that little vanity, has been removed
for safety. This once lively woman who was my wife in another
lifetime lies in morphine sleep, barely recognisable.

*Eileen, Eileen.*

The boys are watching, waiting. Iain, with the knowing but
still slightly unsure air of a student filled with hopes of
becoming a physician, studies his mother's charts. Whatever
technical glyphs he sees there seem to satisfy him. Now
Stephen has to leave, drive back to the airport and pick up
Keiron, complete the reunion, close the circle.

Or so we all think at the time. But we're wrong. Very wrong.
The circle isn't about to be closed just yet.

*Eileen, Eileen.*

She opens her eyes, looks astonished to see me. Maybe she
thinks she's dreaming. The boys have told her I was coming,
but perhaps she's forgotten. Who'd blame her for that? She's
been plunged inside a nightmare and whether she climbs
back out is questionable. She's frail and wasted, floating
between the real world and a morphine variant of it. I may be

a figment. How can she differentiate between what's in her mind and what's not?

She tries tó say my name. She has no voice.

'Don't even try to speak,' I say.

She tries again anyway. What emerges is not even a whisper. Surgeons have been down inside her throat and chest with a laser instrument, burning and cutting at the core of the blockage. God knows what has happened to her vocal chords. She mouths my name. It's the best she can do. I clutch her hand. What to say?

Sometimes at the bedsides of the sick you can be flippant, light – *so what are you doing lazing about like this, you old slacker?* Flippancy depends on the nature of the disease. If this were a routine appendectomy, or a broken leg being mended, an offhand comment might work, bring a small smile, evoke a tiny human connection of some kind. I want to cry really. That's what I want to do. Finding her like this has shipwrecked me. But Eileen doesn't need to see that. And Iain doesn't need it either.

I look into her eyes. Her expression now is one of desperation, and she's frustrated because she can't speak. Her desperation becomes panic, and I lean as close to her as I can in an attempt to catch her words, but it doesn't work. Iain produces a notepad and a felt-tip pen and places it between her thumb and index finger. Then she writes in a manic way, like a medium receiving frenzied messages at a trance. There's an echo of her old energy here, but the words she produces are illegible, tracks that slope off the edge of the page. Iain tries to read them. I try too. The harder we try the more frustrated Eileen becomes because she's not getting through. Eventually the pen just slips out of her limp hand and she quits; we turn the paper this way and that, but we can't read what she's written from any angle.

Iain shrugs, comforts his mother. His manner is soft and caring and at the same time efficient. *You're in good hands* is the message he projects. Soothed, Eileen lies back, looks at me, smiles very slightly, then shapes her mouth into what seems like the words *Thank you*. It takes an enormous effort. She shuts her eyes.

For a while I look at her face. Is she thanking me for making the trip? How can you be as sick as she is and yet feel the need to offer gratitude to anyone? Why isn't she ranting against her illness and plight? Maybe she's just drifting out on the sweet old velvet ocean of morphine and doesn't have the strength for combat. All her gargoyles are dormant for the moment. I kiss her forehead, which is clammy, and linger a few seconds, but she's already been carried away by the docile tides of the drug. Human driftwood. She's exhausted, what little energy she had she burned up in frantic writing. I pick up the sheet of paper. Later I'll try to decipher it.

Outside in the corridor I encounter the doctor who performed the operation on her. He asks if I'm the husband. I tell him I'm the former husband. He's a big man who looks more like a lumberjack than a surgeon, and he's friendly in a professional kind of way. It's hard to imagine this man's life – the bad news he must bring people daily, the fact that his battle against cancer is a deadly slog. I wonder why he chose cancer as his speciality: a loss in his family background somewhere? Or maybe he just likes a good fight, and opponents don't come any tougher than cancer.

He has photographs to show me, colour shots of the work performed on Eileen's windpipe. I see angry-looking red scars against a pink background. These are the marks left by the laser. In an unexpected way they are almost pretty; but so are certain lethal mushrooms. The doctor is saying *this is where we burned* – and I admire the nerve he needs for labouring with such precision in so small an area.

'Her breathing's improved eighty per cent,' he says. 'We're pleased about that. It's a tricky procedure, because there's always a danger you can sever an artery. Instant death . . . I haven't lost anybody that way yet.'

My unasked question hangs in the air. The doctor expects it. You can see it in his face. He's waiting for it because it always comes, it never fails. My attention is drawn briefly to the counter at the nurses' station where a huge box of dough-nuts lies open – yellow and chocolate and white and sprinkled, a deep-fried colourfest of flour and sugar. The night staff must gorge themselves: maybe they don't care about nutrition. Or maybe they eat to pass away the lonely hours of their night watch. It's a kind of sugared escape for them.

I'm aware of Iain standing a few feet away from the doctor and me, as if for some reason he doesn't want to get too close. Perhaps he doesn't want to hear what I'm going to ask or the doctor's response either. Your mother's very ill, you don't want that, you want rah-rah messages, you want physicians to be cheerleaders, bouncing up and down with bright enthusiasm. You want them to be great ball-players. We'll smack death right out of the goddamn field. A homer into the far blue yonder. You wait and see.

I ask The Question. 'What's her prognosis?'

His answer is straight, a doughnut with no frosting. 'It's not great.'

'What time frame are we talking about?'

'A year. Maybe less. Or more.' His voice takes on the qual-ity of an echo. But this is just my jet-lag renewing itself. 'Keep this in mind,' he adds. 'Nobody can predict anything with certainty. Nobody really knows what's going to happen. It's a guessing game.'

I thank him and he turns away and goes down the corridor, taking big steps. Iain has been listening. We walk past the nurses' station. The air smells of fried sugar. Iain is quiet on the way to the elevators. Like Stephen, he wants a miracle. It's not so much to ask, is it? You want your mother made well again. Inside the elevator I want to put my arms around my son and hold him. I want to embrace all three sons at once and tell them Look, it's going to be fine. I promise you that.

But I've made promises to them in the past I haven't kept. I've been careless with their hearts. I know they want to love me without reservation. They want me to be reliable and trustworthy, a solid presence. The problem is a history filled with disappointment and hurt. I don't remember their childhoods with any great clarity, I don't recall a whole bunch of fishing trips, camping, playing ball, doing stuff you're supposed to do with your kids. The starry stuff memories are made of: where is all that?

I look at Iain: he's watching me in a way that is both forlorn and expectant. I put a hand on his shoulder. Unlike his brothers, Iain has never been quite at ease with physical contact. He seems ill-fitted to the world at times, not absolutely connected; a two-prong plug in a three-hole socket. I know so very little about his private life, lovers, friends, how he socialises, if he does even that. I want to say something like *let's just take your mother's situation one day at a time* – a slogan stolen from Alcoholics Anonymous. One day at a time, it's become such a cliché. My sons need more. They need me to be what I've rarely been. A father.

Keiron has arrived and is in the waiting room. I always find a great delight in him. He grasps my hand between his own. The tips of his fingers are callused from guitar-strings. Music is his passion. He's short and his hair is thick and curly; like

Stephen, he gives an impression of physical strength. His face is the kind structured for honesty – it's hard to imagine Keiron managing to conceal any nefarious activity. His expressions give him away all the time, and I don't think he realises it. He projects a kind of innocence. He engages in conversations with total strangers. He has a mysterious knack for somehow giving people a boost. Because he can't make a living playing music, he works part-time as a waiter in an old-money club in Seattle, a role he undertakes with conviction. Off-duty, he dresses like a Seattle musician; no item of clothing matches any other, his shorts hang way below his knees, he wears big black boots.

He's the only son who came to live permanently with Rebecca and me – and Rebecca's daughter Leda – after my divorce. It wasn't an easy situation for either Keiron or Rebecca, but they worked at it. She learned to make allowances for Keiron's natural untidiness, he for her sense of order. It was difficult for Leda too, because she was accustomed to being an only child. But somewhere along the way she realised she'd inherited a trio of brothers – one of whom wasn't just a temporary lodger, he was for keeps.

Now we're together, Iain, Stephen, Keiron and me, and I want to keep this quartet intact as long as I can. I need that second wind you sometimes find on the other side of jet-lag. Things are blurry, though. Any vitality I acquire will be short-lived. I ask Keiron to book us into a hotel for the night, a good one with twenty-four-hour room service. He works the phone in the waiting room, enquiring about room rates, specials, because he knows his way around the hotel industry, the questions to ask desk clerks. He locates a couple of rooms at the Ritz-Carlton, which isn't far from the hospital. My suggestion is that the four of us go there and order food from room service, then Keiron can have one room and I'll sleep in the other, and Iain and Stephen can stay or go as they wish. It's important we have each other in one space for even a brief time, because the shortest amount of time is precious.

Before we leave the hospital, Keiron goes up to look in on his mother. Stephen keeps him company. They want to say goodnight, even if she may not be conscious of their presence: I understand this. Serious illness has never struck this close to them before. I slump in one of the chairs. Here and there in the waiting room people doze or stare into space with worried expressions. Each has somebody sick upstairs. Each has his or her equivalent of an Eileen. We're bonded, even as strangers. I think how, all across this huge continent, all across this vast planet, thousands of people are sitting in waiting rooms similar to this one.

'How long are you staying?' Iain asks.

'A week.' It's not going to be long enough, barely enough time to become acclimatised before I leave again.

'How do you think she looks?' Iain asks.

I don't want to answer the question, so I make a feeble effort to be light-hearted, something along the lines of *she looks like she needs a good meal*. Iain smiles and seems satisfied with this reply, as if this is what he's been waiting to hear all along: there's nothing wrong that proper food can't cure. Malnutrition, that's Eileen's *real* problem. Undernourishment and vitamin deficiency, not malignant tumours. These are the props that support us at bad times. The fragile little railroads we build in our heads so we can move the boxcars of grief around for a while before they have to be unloaded.

The Ritz-Carlton is all airs and graces; reproduction antique furniture, deep rugs, oil paintings. Whoever built the place has made a gallant if misguided attempt to create a new hotel with an old ambiance, but it doesn't have the patina of age. Nothing in this city does. The hotel has a deserted feel to it; I imagine scores of rooms lying empty. July isn't the season for Phoenix, unless you're crazy.

The rooms are adjoining. Keiron picks the one he wants, a mirror image of mine. We order a huge batch of food from room service. Iain is a dedicated carnivore and Keiron hasn't eaten meat – which he calls 'face food' – in years. Iain makes a big play over enjoying his burger, Keiron has a few disgusting things to say about what really goes on inside an abattoir. He piles on gruesome details until I ask him to stop. There's good-hearted banter, a few reminiscences: the infamous time Stephen and Keiron gave me some fish they'd caught, telling me it was rainbow trout, which I cooked and tried to eat – a heap of gristle and bone the kids finally confessed was actually suckerfish, an ugly bottom-feeder with the looks of the Monster from the Black Lagoon. Or our first mind-melting experience of Arizona in the summer of 1976, when we had to stay for a week in a motel with only inefficient and humid swamp-cooling to combat the absolutely devastating heat of Phoenix in August, and I wondered what kind of hell I'd brought my wife and family to live in. The boys remember the long road trip from upstate New York to Arizona (with big family dog), from a smalltown where it snows for six months a year to this desert where you need a magnifying glass to notice the seasons change. They remember an enforced geography lesson, towns with wonderful names – Tucumcari, Amarillo, Albuquerque; the Mississippi River at Memphis, the emptiness of the Texas Panhandle, the dusty dying communities along the old Route 66. Funny, I don't feel like a father – more like some much older brother who's returned to the fold after a series of misadventures.

It's small talk, and it's nice, because we're together, and God knows how often we'll be together this way again. What we don't talk about are the difficult times, the doomed family therapy sessions, separation and divorce, anger and hurt and disappointment, my unpredictability, my absences, the splintering of our lives. This is the bad stuff, and we keep it in our own lockers.

We avoid mention of Eileen also. It's another of those times when we sidestep the hard core of things and enter a world where there's no sickness and a woman isn't fighting for her life in an ICU. We're having a reunion, that's all. A father and his three sons. But then the silences come in slowly and inevitably like a sea fog, and the sound of cutlery stops, and I know we're all looking inward and thinking about Eileen because it's impossible not to. The party sheds its enforced good cheer. Keiron, especially, seems to have subsided into gloom.

Later, a long time later, he'll tell me what's on his mind. 'I looked at her in the intensive-care unit and she just wasn't my mother any more.' He knew, and he resigned himself from that point on to her decline. His decision wasn't pessimistic. He was being, as he saw it, realistic; it was a part of the process of preparation for a world without his mother. He loved her, and she him – undeniably, without qualification, as she loved all her sons; he was the baby, he was the one who was still at home when his older brothers went to school, he was the one who, at the age of four, had vanished the morning after Halloween, pedalling furiously through the neighbourhood on his bright little tricycle, the flap of his Superman cape flying behind him, as he went from door to door searching for a second round of freebies – because he believed the idea of getting candy just by knocking on people's doors was pretty damn terrific and Halloween should be a daily event, maybe even a law on the statute books.

Keiron: the years have tempered this lovely optimism and cheerfulness only a little. He's still undemanding, and laidback, but there's something else about him, something new, maybe Seattle has given it to him – street smarts: it's the only expression I can come up with. He moves differently. His walk has become a kind of lope; a looseness of motion, an ease of gesture. His speech is peppered with the slang of the Pacific Northwest. And none of this seems a deliberate effort to be cutting-edge cool, none of it is studied; it's natural.

I remember the sheet of paper in my pocket and I take it out and look at Eileen's scrambled writing, the snaking lines that run all over the place like a message left in the rain. I think I can decipher, in the midst of all the shapeless words and signs, a single comprehensible message.

It says, *Let me go.*

# 8

*FIGHT fight fight*. This has become the mantra for Eileen. When we visit her in the ICU, this is what we keep coming back to. We say it to her over and over, we whisper it even as she sleeps. In her waking moments she isn't lucid, she still scribbles on her pad and most of what she writes is illegible. She can't speak above a feeble whisper, and none of us understands her.

More people come to visit her. The list of phone messages for her is a long one. She knows scores of people. Friends. People she has helped at the clinic who have become friends. Co-workers. An old friend Dennis Morton, one of the first people we met when we arrived in the United States in 1971, has flown in from Santa Cruz where he runs an alternative supermarket. Dennis the Grocer, who seems never to have aged (I believe a portrait of him, like that of Dorian Gray, hangs in an attic somewhere), is at the hospital constantly. He's easy-going, a superannuated hippie with his hair no longer worn to his shoulders and his huge beard exorcised

years ago. We calculate that maybe seventeen years have
passed since we last met – but that's the touching aspect of
genuine friendships, you fill in the gaps quickly, then you just
get on with things. Time and distance are irrelevant.

Nancy Frick's commitment is unqualified. She's Eileen's
best friend. A tall woman with soulful brown eyes, Nancy has
become a surrogate mother to our sons. She's all things –
switchboard, counsellor, financial advisor, balancer of che-
quebooks, confidante. Sometimes I think she gives too much
of herself because she's not in the best of health and she'll
burn herself out, but I'm not going to tell her so because she'll
swat the suggestion aside like a pestering mosquito. It was
Nancy to whom Eileen turned when she was first diagnosed. It
was Nancy who insisted that Eileen give up her own house and
come and live with her – no easy job, because Eileen's house
had to be emptied and shut down, her possessions scattered,
ferried away by Goodwill, the Salvation Army or just stuck in
dumpsters, a task carried out in the iron-skillet heat of the city
by Iain and Stephen. Keiron had come down from Seattle to
help in the interminable chore of sifting through the belongings of a lifetime and hauling them away. Eileen, who deplored
housekeeping as if it were an experience akin to self-mutila-
tion, had never organised her possessions in any semblance of
order. It wasn't important to her; she could live without noticing disarray.

What to keep? What to throw away? The boxed relics of
her existence, souvenirs, pictures, books, bric-a-brac – in the
end Eileen decided none of it, however precious in sentimental terms, was important enough to keep. Her pets were given
away, and a garage sale raised about $500. In the summer of
1997 her world had been demolished.

Dennis and Nancy and I eat together in nearby restaurants

when we're not visiting the hospital. The food has no taste, it's just fuel; our conversation swirls around the topic of Eileen. Dennis is often emotional. He sees the progress of the disease more clearly than the rest of us; his father died from cancer and Dennis nursed him for a long period. He's travelled this road before. Nancy is stoic, but her stoicism, although admirable and brave, occasionally strikes me as paper-thin, because she's having a hard time looking beyond it and into the future. As we all are.

But as the messages of support pile up, there are moments of hope, because hoping is what humans do – dare we *believe* she can come out of this and that the physician is all wrong? Dare we *believe* there's a turning point somewhere, a junction in the road where the cancer will take a detour and leave Eileen's body? A collective energy keeps hope afloat. But it can only work if Eileen will be combative.

The trouble is, there's nothing pugnacious in her attitude. She isn't attacking her condition. Whatever artillery she might summon is unused and rusting. She lies in bed, attached to a drip, and it's as if, by some contrary act of gravity, her life is draining out of her and rising *up* into the tube that's supposed to be her source of nurture. She seems resigned to her state. Her body has been invaded both by lasers and disease, and her willpower, if it exists after these intrusions, is a flickering thing. I don't want her to fade and die in front of our eyes. But if she isn't there, how can we reach her? If she's absent, float- ing in an unlit space of her own, a black amniotic sac of death, how can any of us get through to her?

Keiron and I move out of the preposterous Ritz-Carlton and into a place called the Embassy, which is close to the hospital; a two-room suite, unpretentious and affordable. The days are becoming hotter. The city is hideously unpleasant, stark and blistering. The sidewalks of Phoenix are empty. The season has created a ghost town. Palm trees survive with more dignity than pedestrians. We crank the air-conditioning up to max, close the curtains, venture out only when we have to.

Between hospital visits, I lie on my bed and smoke. My energy is often zero. The heat makes me lethargic. Keiron talks about his life in Seattle, his band, his stop-gap work as a waiter; he's carved out his own world a long way from the desert. I realise I know nothing about it, I haven't gone there to visit him, I can't see Seattle in my mind's eye or conjure up pictures of Keiron in that city, I don't *see* his life. This makes me uneasy. How has it come to this – that I don't have hard clear images of the life my son lives? I realise it's the same with Iain.

I love Keiron, and I've always thought of us as close, but now I wonder if there's an element of self-delusion in this. If we're as close as I want to believe, why am I not getting pictures of him in a rainy city a thousand miles away? I've never heard his latest band play, never met his girlfriend, don't know what his apartment is like. Do all fathers feel as far removed from their kids as I feel from Keiron? Do they send their sons out into the world and dust their hands and say *Whew, that's my part done, let the kid get on with his life*? I don't want it to be this way. I don't want this pang of anxiety and loss. Suddenly I feel loss spreading everywhere, like some vile plant you can't eradicate because it only grows back again all the more voraciously, and I remember a time years before when Eileen and I were separating, and he said, *'Please don't leave us, Dad,'* and I don't think I've heard anybody sound so sad ever – and when I remember these words now I'm filled with all the anguish and sorrow and terror I felt then.

Was anything in the whole goddamn world worth causing a little boy such pain? I don't know if he has any recollection of

that utterance, or if he's buried it. It's a terrible spook that res-
urrects itself periodically in my memory because I've never
succeeded in interring it. Some things you can't shove deep
into the loam of oblivion and walk away from. Some things
haunt you always. What damage have I done to him? If I ask
him that question directly, I know he'll say there wasn't any
damage. You just weren't like other fathers, but you always did
the best you could, he'll say. *Always, Dad.* Because he wants to
believe it? Because he doesn't want to hurt me? Because he
believes life is better if you have the ability to slough off the
bad parts of your history and go into the future unburdened?

I can't help thinking of the family unit we once were.
Husband wife three sons. How it crumbled and fell apart. A
structure turned to fragments, dust. The stilts were wood-
wormed and then snapped, and the edifice caved in. I
remember that Eileen and I were liberal parents. We didn't
know another way to be. Eileen, if anything, was more lax
than me when it came to discipline of the kids, although neither of us laid down ironclad laws or regulations; but we were
always demonstrative when it came to loving them, we
touched, hugged, we never avoided contact, there was no
standoffishness, no reluctance to reach out to the kids – but
I'm not ready to dwell on the memories of the marriage, not
here in this half-dark air-conditioned room. Later, later. The
only thing that matters right now is Eileen in the present time,
and what we can do for her. If we can do anything.

I say, 'Tell me about Seattle.'

'Come up and visit,' he says. 'See for yourself.'

'I will, I promise.'

'You'll like it there. So will Rebecca,' he says. 'Cool place.
And wet. Phoenix *sucks*.'

I promise him again. And I mean it. He knows I mean it.
I'll find time and I'll go. I must learn that nothing is more

important to children – regardless of their age, six or thirty-
six – than a father who keeps his word.

The Embassy provides breakfast for its guests. Somewhere in
the crowded complex is a breakfast room, a self-service place.
On my fourth morning in Phoenix, while Keiron is still sleeping, I walk through bright sunshine and skirt the edge of the
swimming pool. With the smell of chlorine stinging my nose,
I go in search of this dining room.

Upstairs, I follow a directional arrow. The air smells of
fried bacon and hashbrowns, food I am not allowed to have –
if I adhere strictly to the diabetic diet. (Fibre me to death.
Count my carbohydrates one by one. Hang a crucifix around
my neck to protect me from sugar.) I track the scent to a room
with a buffet and a large dining table, and I serve myself a
little oatmeal, a piece of fruit, blah. I haven't had coffee, I'm a
touch groggy. I carry my plate to a place at the table, half-
noticing that there's a small screen behind me and a projector
at the far end of the table and the other people in the room are
wearing short-sleeved white shirts and neck-ties and little ID
badges. A convention, I think, realtors or insurance guys, and
I dig into the porridge, add a spot of low-fat milk. How good
I am to give my pancreas an easy ride. Take a bow. (I want
bacon and fried eggs, that's what I truly want.)

'What's the subject of your lecture this morning?'

It takes me a few seconds to realise that this question, posed
by a kindly middle-aged fellow in glasses, is directed at me.

'My what?' I ask.

'Just so I can tell the others, give you a little intro, you know
what I'm saying?'

I look around the room. All faces are turned towards me. I
don't know what to say. Lecture? What lecture?

The man says, 'Is there a problem?'

I look a little closer and I see that under the name on the badge – Stanley McGinty – is a set of initials: MPLS. I have a sense of entering a dream. Who is McGinty and what is MPLS and why am I expected to deliver a lecture when all I really want is breakfast before I visit the hospital? Have I perhaps died in the night, and this is a purgatory where you're expected to give talks to a group whose interests you have absolutely no way of knowing, a bunch of keen-eyed eager people whose affiliation lurks behind the acrostic MPLS, which yields no sense? What am I to talk about – veal farming, spelunking, the Highland clearances? And what is the projector for? Am I supposed to have slides to show this bunch?

McGinty is waiting for a reply. This is weird. I look into his eyes and I see concern cloud the friendliness. His smile has become fixed. Maybe this is his worst fear, the guest speaker who freezes. I realise it's a case of mistaken identity, what else, but for a second I'm on the edge of shaking McGinty's hand and telling him I intend to talk in a dynamic way about choux pastry-making or the origins of Braille or the relevance of the crystal in New Age theology, perhaps a deranged synthesis of all three.

I remember suddenly that this isn't the first time I've been confused with somebody else. During the mid 1980s when I lived in Sedona in the Red Rock country of Arizona, I was constantly being mistaken for Dudley Moore. Women would leave scribbled notes under the wipers of my car asking me if I would 'look at a screenplay', phone numbers attached. Once, when I was in a restaurant with Rebecca and some friends, a woman came dashing over to our table and pushed a piece of Indian jewellery into my hand and said, 'This is for all the pleasure you've given me,' and then she rushed away, leaving me to come up with an explanation for Rebecca. Dudley Moore sightings were more common in Sedona than flying saucers for a while. People asked me for my autograph and I always declined, and they'd say things like, 'I understand, you need your privacy, Mr Moore.' I even thought of writing a magazine piece: *My Life As Dudley Moore.* In a way, I enjoyed that time of my pseudo-celebrity. If I'd had a criminal turn of mind, I might have found some way of profiting from it.

And now McGinty is giving me a *second* chance at something few people ever get *once* in their lifetime – *to be somebody else.* He's offering me a new identity, the opportunity to slip out of myself and become this other person, this Breakfast Speaker, informative and witty and charming. I'm grateful to him. He's lightened my heart, unlocked an escape hatch leading from one dimension, where Eileen lies in a hospital and clouds of grief are banked on the horizon, and into another, totally different – a happy place where I don't know anyone with cancer, and nobody's dying, and everything is tickety-boo. And I don't even have to write a word of fiction to reach this halcyon place. I don't have to invent a single character, a line of dialogue, or come up with a plot—

Go for it, Campbell. Shed the skin of your present life. Seize the moment. Goodbye cruel world. Enter McGinty's House of Illusion. One short step and you're in funland. Stephen would do it. He'd revel in this situation. He wouldn't think twice. For him it would be a piece of theatre.

McGinty is becoming suspicious. 'Listen, these folks are growing impatient,' he says. He looks over at the others and makes an exasperated gesture.

Suddenly a guy in a security uniform steps towards the table. He isn't armed, but he carries an evil-looking stick strapped to his belt. 'Is there a problem here?'

How do they know when to ask that question, I wonder. Is it some kind of vibration in the air only security people can detect? I shake my head. 'I'm just having breakfast.'

McGinty makes his eyes narrow and asks, 'Hey, are you really the speaker?'

'I can *speak*,' I say in a vaguely defensive manner.

The security cop leans into my face. 'You don't belong here, do you?'

I'm unmasked. Exposed. Is it something in my eye or the way I'm dressed?

McGinty says, 'If you're not the speaker, you're not entitled to the breakfast.'

The guard immediately whips my cereal away. Shame. Humiliation. The faces that had been watching me with expectation minutes before now look vaguely hostile. *He's an impostor, probably a homeless guy sneaking in for a freebie meal, probably a junkie, I knew it soon as I looked at him . . .* I get up from the table. It's an uneasy moment. The menace and animosity have sealed the door that was my route into another identity. I was given a glimpse of escape and I didn't take it and on top of it all my breakfast has been stripped from me like a medal I wasn't worthy of wearing. I've been deprived of the indulgence of an enticing illusion.

The guard escorts me to the door. I step out of the dining room, which overlooks a central courtyard, blue swimming pool, sunlight on water, the laughter of kids splashing.

'What does MPLS stand for?' I ask.

The guard shrugs. 'Couldn't say.'

All at once I have an overwhelming need to explain things, to put a kind of respectable frame around the fact I mistakenly entered a private dining room and helped myself to breakfast. *It's like this, you see, I'm no breakfast thief, I'm still jet-lagged, my inner clock isn't one hundred per cent, my ex-wife is sick . . .* But the guard has one of those faces that doesn't convey sympathy. Yeah yeah yeah, move it buddy. Fascist, I think. I walk away, aware of him watching me as I go towards the stairs.

Back in our suite where the curtains are shut, Keiron is still asleep. In the bathroom I stare at my reflection in the mirror. The plain truth is: *I look like a bum*. I haven't shaved in days, there are circles under my eyes, and the whites are a little bloodshot, my shirt is crumpled from being stuffed in my bag, my hair needs brushing. I'm the survivor of a wreck. No, I *am* the wreck. *This* is what they allowed into the dining room, this is the figure they permitted to *sit* at the table with his breakfast, this is the guy McGinty imagined was the *speaker*? The only thing the face in the mirror looks capable of talking about is how to panhandle a buck or two for the next bottle of third-rate Muscatel or white lightning. I have seen faces like this at early morning AA meetings in shabby rooms in crumbling downtown areas of major cities, sad guys with tics, trembling fingers, grizzle on their jaws.

I laugh. For the first time in days, I laugh. It's release. It's overflow. It's not exactly a laugh of joy; it comes out of the absurdity of events. I've flown six thousand miles to be ejected from a private breakfast as an impostor, a deadbeat, a poor bastard in need of some chow.

And just for a moment I might have risen to my feet and made a speech. I was on the brink of tunneling my way briefly into another self, a refuge from reality in a charade.

Midday, Keiron and I ride the shuttle bus that travels between the hotel and the hospital. The desert noon light is blinding. At the hospital we go up to the ICU where a young man with curly hair and a clipboard appears, introducing himself as Mark, a hospital social worker. He asks, 'Do you know how the Hospice movement works?'

Hospice movement – what is he *talking* about?

'Eileen has refused further treatment, you see,' he says.

'What do you mean *refused*?'

Mark says, 'Exactly that. She just doesn't want any more treatment. So I need to talk to you about the possibility of getting the Hospice movement involved, and describe the services they provide . . .'

I don't want to hear this. Hospices. Death with alleged dignity, cocktails of cocaine and morphine. I don't understand this kind of talk at all. What has happened here overnight?

Inside the ICU, Eileen is awake and pale. I approach the bed. She raises her face and looks at me and slowly shakes her head. Then she's scribbling on her pad and she writes something that looks like *No More,* and she moves a hand in a small sorry chopping gesture of finality. She's had enough. She doesn't want to go on to the next step in treatment, radiation therapy or whatever else it might be. This is it. It's too painful. The ordeal is too much. *She doesn't want to fight.* She looks at me as if I might be her deliverer, the one who comes with the euthanasia prescription, a little vial of clear liquid I hold to her lips and she drinks, and then she's gone.

There is in her eyes a pleading expression: do it for me, Campbell. Please God, do it for me. I trust you in this. Do what? Hold a pillow over her face until she dies? I sit on the edge of the bed – this is a terrible moment, and I don't know what to say except to chide her gently: *You haven't really thought this through, Eileen. Come on, you're no quitter. You never have been.* I hear my voice, I'm using the bedside tone that comes so automatically during hospital visits. We talk *down* to the sick. Why do we turn them into children? She can't talk back. She doesn't have the strength to write any more either. She's frazzled, her expression is impatient now. There may be anger surfacing.

The doctor comes into the room. He's animated, approaches the bed, takes one of Eileen's hands in his own. 'What's all this stuff people are telling me?' he asks. He doesn't wait for an answer because she can't provide one anyway. 'You want to give up and die? Is that what I'm hearing? Look, you had your chance, Eileen. You had your chance in surgery, and if you wanted to die that was the place to do it. Now you're saying I wasted my time on you? Is that what you're telling me? I put all that work into you for nothing? You know how many years I spent learning how to perform tricky surgery?'

And on. And on.

She stares at him. You can see an interest in her face. Tell me more, Doctor. Swear to me there's life ahead. There's a world where I can live again. Talk to me about how I missed the ferry to the other side. Tell me it isn't time for me to go yet.

'I don't want to hear this kind of crap again,' he says.

He looks at me and smiles. He's delivered his pep talk. I wonder how many times he's done it. I don't doubt for a moment that he cares about his patients, he's dedicated to the maintenance of life. He knows she has a year, maybe less; he's told me so. And yet here he is urging her on, because he can't let a patient choose death, even if – in his professional opinion – there's no great expanse of life left to live. He's an umpire on a high chair, he has judgment calls to make when it comes to living and dying. The ball is never out of the court so long as the patient is breathing and further therapies wait to be tried.

After he's gone from the room I say to Eileen, 'You see. The man says you had your chance and you missed out. Were you listening to him?'

She squeezes my hand. Her grip is a little stronger than I expect it to be. Some of the desperation in her eyes is gone. The stress has lifted, at least for now. I see for the first time how changeable the sickness makes her – up then down, optimism then despair, resolve followed by apathy. Her life is one of sudden emotional extremes, deserts and fertile valleys, flashfloods and desiccated arroyo – landscapes running one into the other without borderlines, without warning signs.

'Don't give up, please don't give up,' I say. 'We need you. Too many people need you.'

She gestures for me to come closer, so she can whisper in my ear.

'This hurts,' she says. 'Oh, this hurts . . .'

And whether she's referring to the pain in her body or her general condition or the fact that she doesn't like to see so many concerned faces inside her room and hovering around her, I don't know, and I can't find out, because she's fallen asleep. I wonder what she's dreaming. I hope it's of some tranquil place, green meadows in sunlight, or a desert under the moon. I hope so.

# 9

I postpone my return trip to Ireland for another seven days. My original intention to stay only one week has been a miscalculation. Had I *really* expected just to fly in, see Eileen get back on her feet in some fashion, then leave again all in the space of seven days – at least three of which had been spent lubricating the clock in my brain? I hadn't been thinking clearly when I left Dublin. But then I had no way of knowing the situation I'd find in Arizona. Rebecca has been urging me to stay. We talk nearly every other day and I've taught her to use e-mail – she's not at ease with computers; I'm never out of touch with her for long. When I speak to her I hear a certain sad note in her voice. Implicitly she's saying, *Stay, you may regret rushing back home.*

By the end of the first week Eileen is recovering slowly from the surgery, if getting your voice back at unexpected moments and being able to spoon down some hospital gruel from time to time counts as recovery. It does, though: each improvement in her condition, however tiny, is an occasion for happiness. Cancer is a wrecking ball, and if you can minimise its destructive path in the smallest way, it's a triumph. Mainly she still speaks in a whisper, and often she's not lucid. She still uses the notepad for most of her communication. She remembers nothing of being moved to the operating room, nothing of writing *Let Me Go* or *No More*. She doesn't recall ever having refused further treatment and initiating a crisis. Later, she'll remember her time in Intensive Care in terms of colours. On the right side of her vision, she saw what she described as the 'strangest shade of grey, swirling. On the left side, there was only black.' She'll also remember a feeling of having been deserted by her God, a state she referred to as 'the ultimate abandonment'.

But now she appears to want to live, and she's already showing signs of impatience about being confined to bed. This is good, this is more like the Eileen of old, these flickers of energy, a light in her eye now and then. She's been moved from the ICU to a regular room. She's very weak. She finds a source of strength in the scores of get-well cards arranged around the room, and cheer from the helium balloon with the funny face, and the odd furry talking toy somebody has attached to the foot of her bed. We spend a great deal of time telling her everything that's happened to her, filling her in on her own history, and what the next step in the procedure is going to be – radiation therapy – and she listens, often with a slightly fearful look: and who can blame her for that? A journey into the unknown, the mysterious destructive powers of radiation. Sometimes she shakes her head as if in a kind of surprise she can't articulate – has this really happened to me? How is it possible?

We talk positively to her at all times, even when she's morphined-out. The theme is upbeat, always upbeat, get well, you can do it. (Goddamn, I sometimes think – this is pantomime, we're going through the motions, she'll never make it. But I shove these discouraging thoughts away. I don't need them.) We stroke her hands, rearrange her clothes and sheets; Iain fusses around, washes her face when she's feeling hot, Stephen makes her laugh even as she implores him not to with hand gestures, because laughing hurts. Iain, I can see, is in his element, nursing, doctoring. I imagine a stethoscope hanging from his neck, the white coat, the little ID badge that reads: Dr I Black, MD. This is all he wants out of life, and so he's buried himself deep in the vault of his studies, and he doesn't come out to participate in the usual student follies, the parties, the girl-hunting, the boozing, the dope. He's in a hurry to reach his destination. Eileen has often told him in the past to relax and unwind, take it easy, life's too short to work so damn hard all the time, but Iain's bought a ticket on a monorail that only stops at Degree Central.

I speak to Eileen sometimes about the old days. Glasgow, London, New York. Do you remember that snobby tea-room on Sauchiehall Street? What was it called? Do you remember that crazy landlady I had in London and the time somebody strangled her pet pigeons and she blamed me? And what about that horrible arse-freezing town with the nuclear energy plant where we lived in upstate New York, a burg that had about half a million bars and everybody was always either stoned or inbred or maybe suffering brain deterioration from the bad energy buzzing out of the plant? She nods to each of these questions: memories have some delights. You can escape through them, reassure yourself, wallow in ancient comforts the way you might in a shoebox of treasured family photographs.

Iain, Stephen, Keiron, myself, and Nancy Frick form the core of regular visitors: Dennis has had to return to Santa

Cruz where his grocery business is going downhill towards bankruptcy. People with Dennis's hippie background don't always make good businessmen, and he's had problems with a partner he took on board. He'd rather read poetry and play jazz on Santa Cruz public radio, where he has a weekly programme

Keiron, who can't get any more time off work, has to go back to Seattle. I don't go to the airport to see him catch his plane. Farewells are tough at any time, but especially now. I remember being at Shannon with Stephen only a month ago, I can't keep doing this, putting my sons on aeroplanes, sending them off through space. Keiron will be in touch continually, it's just that he's not absolutely sure when he'll be back – it may be a week, even longer. He has to come to some arrangement with his employer. I dislike those sad little cameos of partings in airports. Something in the atmosphere at the departures gate acts as a licence for otherwise undemonstrative people to display public emotion; I'll come unglued if I have to hold him and tell him goodbye. Also, I have a feeling that whatever fortitude I possess I'll need for the eventual time of my own departure. Only a week away now.

There's no point remaining in the Embassy without Keiron, and I really don't want to be alone, so Iain offers me the spare room in his apartment, which is in the southern part of Tempe, one of Phoenix's satellite towns. A gluttonous city, Phoenix feeds off the communities of Scottsdale, Glendale, Tempe, Mesa. Bloated, it lies spread across the Valley of the Sun and the hum of its freeways never ceases. For all its size, it seems to me without heart or soul, homogenised beyond blandness. This is one boring city.

The only reason I can see for its existence is that masochists are drawn here to broil themselves; human crackling. They come because they are sun fetishists attracted by the alleged 'laid-back' Southwestern lifestyle, which strikes me as a massive con perpetrated by realtors and Chamber of Commerce types with homes for sale and empty business premises in need of buyers. Come on down to the desert, they cry, these suntanned men with their stetsons and bola ties, these sharp-nosed real-estate beagles in their tan blazers, these commission-hunters and investment bankers and assorted dealmakers. Come on down, enjoy the calm unhurried life of the great Southwest.

The newspapers are slab-thick with get-rich-quick business opportunities and homes you can walk into with few formalities – No Money Down! Mortgage Assumable! Glossy C-of-C brochures depict barbecues in back yards cluttered with palm trees and people in Bermudas and luscious golf courses kept wondrously green by water diverted from the seriously overworked Colorado River. Hurry. Your future is waiting. Hurry. Before the Colorado dries up.

Calm? Laid-back? No, it is as frantic as any other big city. It's a sell-sell-sell US smalltown that outgrew its humble origins as a watering hole in the desert. The freeways are clogged. Drivers are hot and angry and pressured. They drive with hostility and paranoia: it is Los Angeles in the desert.

Along Camelback, one of the main thoroughfares in Phoenix, is what I think of as the true essence of the city: Car Corridor, one auto dealership jammed alongside another, block after block, thousands of cars, practically a small *city* of cars, where salesmen circle like sharks and offer deals that only lunatics could turn down – we finance, bankruptcy or bad credit or NO credit, hey, no problem, sign here! Cars and cars and cars in all colours and shapes. Bunting hanging everywhere, and advertising blimps in the sky. No car is unaffordable. Just take a look, buddy. *Like the '92 Caddie? Boy, is she loaded or is she loaded? I figure we can work out a sweet deal. No sweat.*

But everything is sweat here. The air is putrid and the water supply is low and the sun scalds and people are thirsty and they sweat. I imagine millions of gallons of water coming through shower heads or flushing toilets; and more millions of gallons frittered away in sprinkler systems that keep lawns looking, yeah, *real* nice – except that grass in the desert always looks fake to me, spraypainted in place.

I have no idea what Eileen enjoyed here. The sun? The desert terrain – which I find brown and deadly, all hidden snakes and invisible spores? I brought her here and then eight years later I left her – but what kept her? It's a mystery. Maybe she felt an affinity for the atmosphere; after the hard rains of growing up in gritty Glasgow, perhaps she needed this monotonous blue furnace. Or maybe the desert gave her a sense of spirituality the way it does to some people, who find self-transformations in all that sky and space and shimmering heat on hazy distant horizons. I know she has mild New Age inclinations, nothing far-out, no weird affinities, no spaceships coming to disgorge beautiful people from distant places to teach our species how to live, no Indian guides capable of shapeshifting. She's a little too sensible to subscribe to that kind of thing. She combines the practicality of her two heritages – the Jewish and the Scots.

Iain, who can't afford school tuition if he moves out of Arizona, dreams of rainy cool places. His apartment, where I take my suitcase after Keiron leaves, is dark, shades always drawn, the main light source located inside a large fish tank. It's comfortable, and I have the place to myself much of the time; Iain is often in class at ASU. Too often.

Although Eileen is returning to some semblance of life, in truth it's a counterfeit thing, the play of hand-shadows on a wall. Even if by some miracle they could eradicate the cancer from her body, she'd live with the fear that it might lurk – a sub-microscopic malingerer ready to strike again – in some deep recess of her system. And this is hard to take.

I think of my father, who died of the same disease in 1982 when I was in America, and my visa had expired, I had no green card, I was an illegal and I couldn't leave the country because I would have no easy way of getting back in again. And this is hard to take as well – that I was absent from his dying, that his death was borne by my mother and sister without me; that my last conversation with him, conducted by telephone, was inconclusive, his speech breathless.

*Are you doing okay, Dad?*

*Fine, just fine.* (He can hardly talk above a pathetic whisper: like Eileen's, his voice seems to come from the far end of an abandoned railroad tunnel.)

*I wish I could come over.*

*Ach, don't worry about it. I'll be fine.*

Even as he was dying, we were trapped in a revolving door of a conversation. And I missed his funeral. I missed being there to comfort my mother and my young sister Joy.

I seek numb. I court numb. I would lay palm fronds down in the procession of numb to welcome it. But it has a fragile crust and you keep falling through into a place where emotions come at you like torpedoes – neglected torpedoes, their navigational equipment suspect after years of inactivity. I haven't examined my own heart often enough. I haven't submarined down into the depths of myself and my motivation as I might have done. I try to blame this half-examined life on a couple of factors. The first is that I write fiction, a selfish occupation; I'm happier dealing with the emotions of made-up people, figments I've invented. The second is cultural. I come from a race of people – hardy and northern, flinty Presbyterian souls – who for the most part have always been, just like my father, suspicious of self-analysis. If you had soul-searching to do, you did it in church. Lift up your voice, and you lift up your heart. If you had emotional problems, you talked with your GP. All that psychoanalytical guff was for the weak and the artsy-fartsy. Don't waste your bloody time. Or your money.

Eileen's disease is changing everyone around her, including me.

# 10

Eileen's release from hospital is imminent. She has very little money of her own, but her state medical insurance allows her to be transferred to an after-care unit, a nursing home. She's nervous about being moved. She's become cocooned in her hospital room. We all reassure her – *look, love, you're getting out of this damned hospital and these after-care places are OK and in any case it's only for another week, ten days tops, and then you're free* . . . She tries to grasp this idea of going out into the world again, beyond the boundaries of hospitals and nursing homes. And maybe she tries to imagine a reality like the one she knew before she was sick. Going back to work, driving her car, looking after herself, doing the simple things she's always taken for granted – a shower, clipping her toenails, applying a little makeup. (Her skin colour is a kind of hospital puce. She looks heart-breakingly feeble some days.) I'm not sure she believes that kind of life will be possible again. She's thinking of radiation therapy, there's a whole course planned, and it's iffy, an imprecise science, it can do more damage than good: she *knows* all this.

'You can get through it,' we tell her. 'You can do anything you set your mind to.'

We have become a Greek chorus of sorts by this time; but instead of lamenting, we're uplifting, we're encouraging. Stephen and Iain are remarkable in attentiveness to their mother, how they anticipate her needs. Wash her face. Her hands. Make sure she brushes her teeth. This is what love comes down to in the end – an indestructible emotion illness can only strengthen.

There's no vanity. These boys don't care what their mother looks like, that she needs a decent haircut, that her face is thin and sunken and she's the colour of a lettuce, that she's changed, her voice hasn't come back properly, her state of mind is delicate, her body host to viciously unpredictable cells – this is still their mother and by God they love her, and *nothing* can ever change that. And she returns the love with a flash of old humour; one day she scribbles something on her notepad and holds it up for us to see. She's written BLACK POWER. Black, the family name. I wrote my first few novels under my real name of Campbell Black, before I assumed the pseudonym Armstrong. Black Power is herself, the kids – and me. We can do anything! There's nothing we can't defeat! You're a winner, Eileen. You'll pull through this shit!

Iain's worried about nursing homes; he's heard stories of helpless bedridden people being robbed in these after-care places, sometimes beaten. He wants to investigate the two nursing homes for which Eileen is eligible. He's determined to make sure they satisfy him before he places her in their care, and he takes control of this situation. He's in his milieu again, he's worked part-time in these places as a paramedic, he knows what to look for, the questions to ask.

So, on another hot Phoenix morning, Iain, Stephen and

myself visit one of these homes. Iain says, 'I'll do the talking,
OK?'

'It's up to you,' Stephen says.

The facility is close to downtown. It's a brick-built place of
a depressing functional nature, a concrete slab parking lot, a
couple of trees. Iain scopes it out before we go inside, like a
thief casing a joint. He's looking for security cameras, evidence of alarm systems. Inside, there's an institutional scent in
the air – that slightly bland combo of floor polish, soap and
indeterminate cooking smells. There's a certain bustle up and
down the central corridor – nurses, paramedics, janitorial staff.
Iain approaches the desk in a brisk manner. He explains to the
receptionist that he's thinking of placing his mother here. A
pleasant woman, the Assistant Director, is summoned; she's
blond and friendly and bubbly, ready to answer any questions
Iain has.

He goes into action at once. 'I want to know your policy
concerning personnel,' he says. 'Do you run checks on them
for criminal records?'

*Criminal records*; I haven't thought about this. Nor would I.
It's Iain's way. In his mind I am sure he imagines the possibility of a psychotic male nurse abusing helpless female patients,
or his sick mother at the mercy of a thief with a knife at her
throat.

The woman answers calmly. 'All our personnel are thoroughly checked before we employ them.'

'Out of state too?' Iain asks.

'Of course. We don't restrict our background checks to
Arizona.'

Iain seems halfway satisfied. 'It's just that I need to know
my mother's going to be safe here.'

'We take every precaution,' the woman says. 'I can assure
you of that.'

And now we get the guided tour of the facility. Iain is vigilant, as if his eyes are on retractable stalks. I have never seen him this wary, this *careful*, before now. He might be the Inspector-General of Arizona Nursing Homes, a watchful bureaucrat sent to look for misdemeanours, broken rules. We see the rooms, the recreation area, dining-room, bathrooms. Iain seems to be working from some invisible check-list. I can hear him tick items off in his head. In the big stainless-steel kitchen area I have an unexpected flashback – I'm whisked down through time to school in Glasgow, and I'm inside the dining hall, and there are great metal tubs of dry mashed potatoes and some kind of swill masquerading as gravy, and meat that came from the bones of an unidentifiable animal and peas – dear God, the *peas*, were they ever really *peas* in a *pod*? – cooked into a gelatinous mass. This is how communal kitchens affect me.

I step out into the corridor. *Eileen hasn't much of an appetite at the moment anyway*, I think. *Just as well*. Strange the way thousands of miles and forty-something years collapse in an instant, and I'm a kid in a school dining hall in the east end of Glasgow, not a grown man in a nursing home in Phoenix. Another piece of escapism, a way out of this unhappy situation and back to a time when such trivia as school food was *important*.

The tour continues. The patients are a mixed lot. There are terminal cases attached to machines, people recuperating from illnesses, accident victims on the mend. Young, middle-aged, elderly. The place is beginning to grind down on me – and yet it isn't unpleasant, it's clean, bright, the staff are friendly. It's still an institution, that's the problem, and it saddens me to think of Eileen coming here. And for how long? Nobody has been very specific about that. Nurses don't know. Physicians can't tell you for sure. Everything hinges on ignorance and uncertainty: only the cancer is real.

*

Outside, Iain says, 'It felt okay. What do you think?'

'It seems fine,' I answer. Fine as such a place can be.

Stephen says the same. We decide there's no point in visiting the other nursing home on our list, which is located in a part of the city the kids don't like.

Later, Iain calls the hospital social worker to make arrangements, and next day Eileen is brought to the nursing home by ambulance. And I realise now, probably for the first time really, that my spell in Arizona is coming to an end. I have a couple of days, no more. I can't cancel my flight again. I have another life to live.

I'm depressed – even as I'm relieved by the prospect of escaping this heat. And, to be honest, the sickness too, I have to run from that, I've been living with it daily to the point where my scalp feels like the tightly drawn skin of a drum, and I'm not sleeping well because I'm stressed, powerless, I can't do a goddamn thing to help Eileen back to good health—

But this is selfish thinking. This isn't taking into account Eileen's needs. She has to live with her wasting illness twenty-four hours a day. And the boys, I'll be leaving them also – and they'll have to contend with their mother without me.

I'll be six thousand miles away in Ireland. I have to reconcile myself to this fact. I'm going home. I have another life.

Eileen will need an apartment when she's released from the nursing home, whenever that will be. Stephen has already decided he'll live with her; his marriage is still ruptured and he hasn't had time to think about the extent of the damage to it, and so it makes sense to share a place with his mother. He'll also be on hand to help her. He and I go looking for a place.

Phoenix is overloaded with apartment complexes. Motionless banners outside these complexes proclaim all kinds of offers. FIRST MONTH FREE. NO SECURITY

DEPOSIT REQUIRED. RENT BY THE WEEK, THE MONTH, THE YEAR. CABLE READY. We look at a few. Some are hideous, screendoors busted and hanging at weird angles, stained carpets, appliances that look about as safe as electric chairs. Some places have decidedly dodgy-looking tenants, shifty guys in shades lounging around soda machines and smoking in the sunlight as if they're waiting for dark before their nefarious work really begins. Others have swimming pools so loaded with chlorine your skin would be peeled off. And others still are only a rung up from slumdom.

A few upscale ones amuse me, because they're not only renting apartments, they're trying to promote a way of life – the girls who greet you in the rental offices are chirpy and healthy and sun-tanned, and *muscular*, and talk about the, like, oh-wow, high-tech gymnasium facilities in the complex; they all sound as if a looped tape has been surgically inserted into their heads. I wonder if at night they keep hearing the same spiel in their brains. Does it follow them into their dreams? The girl at the Brandywine apartment complex who answers the phone each time with the sing-song phrase, 'Hi, it's a wonderful day at the Brandywine, how can I help you?' – has she been tampered with? A synapse altered by corporate fiat? *It's a wonderful day at the Brandywine*. She makes Brandywine sound like goddamn Xanadu. It could be pissing down, or hurricanes tossing Winnebagos in the sky, or hissing fissures appearing in the earth, and it would *still* be a wonderful day at the Brandywine. And she looks like she means it. With her straight white teeth and pert little mouth, she'd *never* lie to you, would she?

Eventually we find an apartment we like. The manager of the complex tells us proudly it's one of the oldest in Phoenix, goes all the way back to 1964. 'They don't build 'em this way any more,' she says. 'Sound-proofed and made to last.' In fact it's a nice place, old shade trees, a series of little courtyards, a swimming pool, and buildings that have an air of permanence to them – rare in the Valley of the Sun, where everything seems to have been thrown together with obsolescence in mind.

'Mom'll like this,' Stephen says. This is what's important to him: Eileen's environment. Nothing else matters. He explores the place with a look of concentrated concern.

I walk through the empty rooms. A kitchen. A sitting room. A bedroom. It's shadowy and cool. It could be comfortable. There are no stairs to climb. There's a small fenced patio area.

'It needs furniture,' I say. 'You'll especially need a sofa bed for the living room.'

'No problem. We'll hit the second-hand stores,' Stephen says. He's suffused with confidence. An important chore has been accomplished: he's found an apartment. The breezy tone in his voice is that of a young man who doesn't understand the meaning of the word obstacle.

'Then you ought to take it, if you like it. You'll be living here too.'

He decides to rent it. Fills in the forms, leaves a deposit. And so now we have a place to bring Eileen when she's sprung from the after-care residence. This place she has never seen before will be home.

For how long?

Eileen's room at the nursing home is small. Her bed is located next to the window; the other bed in the room is occupied by a very old woman with sparse white hair and whose skin is covered with liver-spots, brown archipelagoes on a pale map. She sleeps all the time. She's dying. Checking out. She looks as if half of her has already gone on ahead to reconnoitre The Beyond. This isn't good company for Eileen. What Eileen needs around her is life, vivacity. She needs plants and flowers, and people who can talk with her.

She has her own sink and mirror. Iain has rigged up a small portable fan at the side of her bed, because the air-conditioning in the room isn't very effective. Sun beats against the window beside the bed all day long, and heat seeps through the walls. Her toiletries are lined up on a table beside her. Hairbrush and comb, toothbrush and toothpaste. The small inconsequential stuff of her life is gathered around her. What is it about these tiny possessions that makes me melancholy? Perhaps I think ahead, I make a leap into the future, to that time when Eileen will cease to exist – and all that is left will be her stuff, her things, the belongings of the dead. And these abandoned items will vibrate, however thinly, with the last dying energy of their owner—

No, quit, these are the fancies of sadness. They come from saying goodbye. Not knowing when I will see her again. Or if I will see her again. Or never. Never is the kind of word that lances the heart. Sucks the breath out of you.

Never is the most goddamn final word of all.

I sit on the edge of the bed and hold her hand. She looks bright-eyed today; she's lucid. I take her fingers between my own. She doesn't seem scared. For the first time since I arrived she has an air that is almost one of confidence. I tell her about the apartment. I describe it, and she listens, looking pleased. There has also been some talk about her brother Sydney coming to visit in the near future, and this cheers her too.

I don't know how to remind her that I'm leaving.

But I don't have to. She whispers, 'You won't be here in the morning.'

No, I won't. I have a flight. I must go. I have a ticket and a departure time.

'You helped me,' she says. She hasn't lost her Glasgow

accent after almost twenty years in the United States. There's the occasional little American twang, an American expression or two. But she's still southside Glasgow. 'You really helped me by coming.'

'I'll come back,' I say.

'I know you will.'

And I will, I most surely will. All the promises I have broken in my life, all the good intentions shattered – this time I give my word and I mean it.

'Thank Rebecca for me,' she says.

'Thank her?'

'For sending you.' And she smiles.

I kiss her forehead. She releases my hand. I walk outside, I don't look back.

In the morning Stephen and Iain drive me to the airport. I want to get away quickly, no lingering, no drawn-out good-byes. I pass through the metal-detector and I'm gone, and once again I don't turn to gaze back. I can't bear the way people dwindle in your line of sight, the strange harrowing irrational fear that maybe this is the last time you'll ever meet – your plane will plunge into the sea, or somebody will have an accident on the freeway on the way home from the air-port: the last two weeks have topped up the compartments where apprehension is stored.

In one hour I will be five hundred miles away, heading east toward Atlanta. In five hours I'll be over the Atlantic.

Quick, walk quick, move, get away. Quick. Quicker now. Don't turn. Your heart is crashing.

# 11

It's a warm July morning in Dublin, and sunny – a different sun from the American Southwest, this one almost benign, an older sun with less fire in its belly. I'm glad to be back. I feel weird, schizophrenic, part of me in Arizona still, the other in Ireland. It's as if I split into two people somewhere close to the eastern seaboard of the United States and I can't put this pair of eggshell selves back together again.

I take a taxi from the airport into the city of Dublin, where I meet Rebecca at her daughter Leda's house in Rathmines. Old streets and houses, Georgian squares, grubby old Dublin – how wonderfully different from Phoenix it is. I'm happy to see Rebecca again, and Leda, and her two small children. Leda has always had a good relationship with Eileen. Eileen accepted Leda into her family, just as Rebecca accepted Keiron and Stephen and Iain – although he took longer – into hers. During times when Leda was in Arizona, she often visited Eileen. And on one scrap of paper written in a crazed state in Intensive Care, Eileen scrawled the words LOVE LEDA. So there's a relationship between them, and I know that Eileen's condition upsets Leda – even if, like Iain, she plays poker with her feelings at times, and you can't always read from her face what's in her heart.

All I want now is to drive down the country, go home, sleep in our own house. I want the quiet of the bog, the great impenetrable silences of the night. I bring Rebecca up to date on the health situation as we drive south from Dublin, but she knows Eileen's condition in any event from the e-mail flow of information. We pass through small towns – Kildare, Mountrath, Borris-in-Ossory. Sometimes in winter these are the drabbest places imaginable, coffin towns. Today in bright sunlight they're almost festive. Good to see greenery again, lush and vibrant. Good to see grey stone walls and small shops, many with their old-fashioned signs and family names. Good to be plugged into history again, that feeling of continuity. And good to be with Rebecca, even if I still have the dry taste of Phoenix in my mouth.

It's another world I've come from; and yet it's not.

I want to sleep for a very long time.

But I wake early, my internal clock awry. Daylight is sneaking through a space in the heavy shutters of our bedroom. I wander the house, try not to wake Rebecca, go downstairs, make coffee. Then I sit in my office, sip the coffee, watch the early light of day spread across the fields. Stephen's presence still hangs in my room. When I switch on my computer I hear the message he recorded the night before he left back in June. *What are ye gonna do?* posed in the heavy Scots accent he affected at the time. I think of him now, I wonder where he is at this moment, it's evening in Arizona, maybe he's at the nursing home with his mother, I don't know. And the night he was born comes back to me – a vivid picture; an unforgettable one. Serious, surreal, shattering, all of these.

If Iain was an insomniac child who couldn't be bribed to sleep with warm milk or pacifiers dipped in honey, and who screamed inexplicably at all hours – I couldn't cope, I wasn't ready for a screeching child – Stephen was the complete opposite. He didn't wake except to be fed, and then immediately went back to sleep again. He was born in the bedroom of a small house Eileen and I had bought after my graduation from Sussex and our move back to London. In 1968 I'd found work in publishing as assistant editor to a man called Tony Godwin, a brilliant but erratic editor, volatile, given to book-throwing tantrums, at the house of Weidenfeld & Nicolson.

The job was fun but often frustrating, because I was sometimes stuck between the conflicting demands of Godwin on the one hand, and George Weidenfeld on the other – the sharp wiry imp here, the doe-eyed cardinal there. I was also a little bored by some of the books Weidenfeld was bringing into the house and giving me to edit – books written by friends in high places, or the offspring of friends in high places, the memoirs of this peer or that one; social rank and influence was of more interest than ability, it seemed. I lasted one year at this firm – I loved Godwin, but not his histrionics – before I moved on to accept an editorial job at Granada, which was run by Sidney Bernstein. The interview consisted of me presenting myself in Bernstein's office in Soho and of him saying, 'Well, let's have a look at you then,' and that, puzzlingly, was that. I was hired and placed in charge of an imprint called Rupert Hart-Davis and given an expense account and told to acquire books.

These were the dear long-gone liver-damaging days of

legendary lunches, three hours, four, stumbling from restaurant to drinking club; certain literary agents enjoyed these long boozy afternoons, although I don't remember any great books being acquired as a result of them. I do remember, however, passing many afternoons in an air of befuddlement – alcohol was everywhere, an intrinsic part of the business then. You just never said no to a drink. It was a heresy. I was learning more about booze than book publishing. Campari or negroni before lunch, two bottles of wine during, a brandy after, and then perhaps cold lager at a place like the seedy old Capricorn Club or the Tattie Bogle in Soho.

I was on the slipway. I missed appointments. After work, I drank until closing time with authors. I was always late to arrive at the office in the mornings. Granada was a place of extraordinary tolerance for its employees' peccadilloes. It had to be, because it housed people of talent but also of uncertain temperament. Carmen Callil, who worked in publicity, and would later create her own publishing house and become generally famous in literary circles; the bright Tony Richardson, now dead, who established an imprint called Paladin, which was later run by Sonny Mehta, now head of Knopf; the amazingly eccentric, self-destructive editor Michael Dempsey, a wild character, also dead, in slightly puzzling domestic circumstances – changing a lightbulb, he slipped and fell; Patrick Janson-Smith, PR assistant, later to create an imprint called Black Swan. I revelled in the atmosphere of Granada.

God knows how many times I disappointed Eileen by not coming home at the promised hour, or sometimes turning up with a drunken writer in tow – somebody I could use as an excuse or a shield if she was angry with me. And she had every right to be angry at times, and yet what I recall most was not anger but a look of hurt that would always yield before too long to forgiveness. I pored through crappy manuscripts at home for hours when all I wanted was to write my second novel – the first, a dark comedy, had appeared to moderate acclaim and reasonable sales. I edited books over which I fell asleep, I was juggling too much, I had financial pressures, mortgage, car, the usual: in Eileen's eyes, I was a perfect candidate for forgiveness and understanding.

I had some half-assed notion that the birth of the second child would restore my equilibrium, balance the vessel of myself. I saw signs about my behaviour that were disturbing even to me – but at that time they were located on a far horizon, out of focus, blips on a radar screen. The marriage itself still seemed basically solid. And the new baby would reinforce it.

I wanted to be present at the birth. This was important, the participation, seeing the emergence of the baby. The pregnancy had been a relatively easy one for Eileen, and I hadn't been nervous – at least not until the moment when her waters broke and I had to telephone the midwife (this was the practice of the time if you had your child at home). The midwife was understanding; she'd seen me thousands of times – apprehensive fathers-in-waiting, troubled by phantom worries, saying such things as *maybe the doctor should be here, maybe you'll need help.* But the only help the midwife needed was me to hold Eileen's legs apart, which I did; Eileen, in the hard pain of labour, was taking gas and air and telling me, in the intense manner of someone stoned, that it was important we love our neighbours, especially the irksome Valerie who lived in the house next door and whom Eileen couldn't stand. *Valerie means well,* she said. *Look at the world from her point of view.* Although this babble was amusing, I was more concerned with the task of keeping Eileen's legs apart, because she had a tendency to want to slam them shut, so I needed to use my strength, and all the while Eileen was continuing her Love-Thy-Neighbour sermon.

And suddenly there was the head of a baby—

This will never leave me. This is one picture that will never go away. I was flattened by the sight, shocked, enchanted, bewitched, privileged – I watched the child emerge and the midwife held it and said *you have a son, congratulations.* This tiny creature, this small crying boy: how had Eileen and I contrived to produce this living breathing heartbeating little person? It was impossible, some kind of miracle. I shook, I couldn't keep my hands still, I was beset by awe and something I can only describe as a feeling of unworthiness – this pure child, this innocent thing, what right did I have to be its father? I drank too much, I wasn't a great husband, I couldn't possibly be the father this child deserved. He needed somebody better. He needed a reliable man. Somebody strong. I would love him, of course I would, but love wasn't enough on its own – on and on, this head-spinning sense of my own lack of value, this fusillade of – what? guilt?

The midwife asked me for some sheets of newspaper. I found them. She wrapped something inside the paper and told me to burn it in the yard behind the house. It took me a couple of moments to understand she was giving me the afterbirth, the placenta wrapped in the *Guardian.* Burn it, yes. Take it outside, yes. Strike a match, fine. Will do. I was a zombie. I was still trembling. Outside, on an April night and starry over London, I struck a match and I cried and I lit the newspaper and I found I couldn't stop crying, *Jesus Christ what was wrong with me?* The paper sparked in my hand. I dropped the smoking papers with the placenta on to the ground. The fire went out, the afterbirth hadn't caught flame, hadn't even smouldered. *Stop fucking crying*, I told myself. *Stop it.* I looked down at the scorched paper and the afterbirth visible through the half-burned sheets. What now? What do I do with this now?

I went back inside the house and said, 'It won't burn.'

The midwife said, 'Fine. Then bury it.'

'Bury it?'

'Use a spade or something.'

Eileen, still a little zoned, was holding the silent sleeping baby.

I went back outside, found a spade, dug a small hole. I shoved the placenta and blackened sheets of paper inside and filled the hole. Finished. Buried. Why hadn't the midwife suggested that in the first place? Didn't she know that after-birth didn't catch fire easily? I wiped my eyes with my sleeve. I stood very still. An aeroplane passed overhead on its descent to Heathrow. The sky roared. I listened to the beat of my heart. Be still, I told myself. Be very still. Breath slowly. Relax. A new life lies in your wife's arms in the upstairs bedroom of this suburb in North London. Celebrate that. Let that be your joy. A new baby. A second son.

And then my attention was drawn to something furry snuffling nearby. I heard the unmistakable sound of an animal pawing earth in a frantic way. Our dog! Our goddamn dog! She'd dug up the placenta and was running all around the back yard with the damn thing hanging from her jaws. I gave chase, round and round in circles, *come on, doggie, be nice, give me back the afterbirth, please, good doggie*. But it was rich in goodies, heavy with protein, meaty, a wonderful find for a scavenging dog. I chased and chased and finally cornered the animal and seized the placenta from her mouth and dumped it in the trashcan and slammed the lid down hard and thought: Why hadn't the midwife suggested putting it in the trash in the first place instead of asking me to flambé the fucking thing?

I walked back indoors, breathless.

'Everything fine?' the midwife asked.

'Everything's taken care of,' I said.

I looked at Eileen, who was half-asleep, drained, her hair damp with sweat, her face slightly stressed. The baby had been placed in a crib beside the bed and wrapped in blankets. I gazed at him. Only his face was visible. I thought: I love you. I'm your father, and I'll always love you and I'll look after you. And I'll always love your mother too.

And nothing will alter that.

I remember Stephen's birth now as I sit in my office in Ireland with daylight filling the fields. I have work to do, a book to write, but somehow the urgency recedes, another novel, does the world need another novel anyhow? It seems unimportant to me at this time. The mood will come back, but not immediately. I'm distanced a little from the ambition that has always fueled me, which is to write – but sometimes I look back and I think, Christ, I've written hundreds of thousands of words, who knows how many, and have any of them made any difference to the world? Maybe a little entertainment to some – but entertainment can be had with less effort from TV or cinema. I know what this is, this mood, I'm going through a gloomy phase that's connected with Eileen's condition, which has put in question the value of my own life's work, and whether it's been worth all the countless solitary hours spent in front of typewriters or computers, the ache in the shoulders, the deteriorating eyesight, the struggle for a word, the key to a character's motivation, an image. What the hell does it matter to the reader anyway if I pick the right image or if I leave it out entirely? Is it going to ruin the narrative if I describe a rainy day as 'smelling like a damp dog' or if I just leave it out? Who cares? Who *really* cares?

I hate this mood. I think of how I'd feel if I had cancer instead of just this general existential malaise, this mid-life drift. I need to put these feelings in perspective. *Eileen has the real ailment, not me.* In the days that follow, I ease back into writing a novel. I like the theme, I like the tension, I have sympathy for the central character. Normally, this would be pleasure – but I'm distracted, I'm sending e-mails to my sons asking about Eileen's condition, and the messages I get back are that she's trying naturopathic treatments, scary-sounding remedies from Mexico or France or Canada. She's also been seeing some kind of faith healer.

Iain has no sympathy for such 'practitioners'. He calls all alternative medicine 'naturopathic homeopathic freakopathic crap' and he doesn't want Eileen to get involved with it. He'd like to protect her from charlatans such as the so-called 'healer' who came to the apartment one time and made some melodramatic passes with his hands up and down her spine, so banishing forever the evil of cancer. *Like hell.* Iain loathes anything that strays from the straight and narrow of conventional treatments; everything must conform to the textbooks. Comprehensible, scientific, nothing mystical, nothing that hasn't been thoroughly researched and tested. And yet he'd gladly embrace a 'miracle' if one came to his mother's rescue: the paradox of the physician faced with the dying of a loved one – in the end, science can go take a flying leap off a high rocky promontory if an off-the-wall cure turns up, some last-minute supernatural occurrence, say, or the crushed roots of a rare Amazonian poppy whose properties eradicate the disease.

I receive mail from Eileen herself. It's optimistic. She says she has 'hunger pangs', which she considers a good sign. She is working on 'visualisation' to diminish the tumours. She tells me a dream she recently had: 'I looked up at the sky and saw some light clouds. Behind the clouds I saw lightning bolts.

# 12

SYDNEY, Eileen's brother, has been a widower since 1977. He's lived in the same tenement flat on the south side of Glasgow for most of his adult life. His son, Brian, lives at home; his daughter, Brenda, has married and moved a few miles away. Sydney's trade is a hard one; he sells all manner of goods – toys, key-rings, souvenirs, fad items, aspirins, Bandaids, tights, hairspray, stationery, footballs – to general stores and newsagents. His work takes him all over Glasgow, and beyond, to such outlying towns as Greenock, Troon, Largs. He's been in this business for years. The market is up and down, as markets usually are. Sydney's is down more than up. He's tired much of the time, he's overweight, his circulation could be better. He loves Eileen, and the news from the United States has been depressing him. He's planning a trip to see her.

For most of his career his suppliers, mainly Asian wholesalers, were clustered in the Gorbals, a slum district just south of the Clyde with the worst housing record in the United Kingdom. Each day for years he'd driven its dreary streets, picking up his stock at one or another of the warehouses, ill-lit places where shelves were stacked with inexpensive toys, soaps, shampoos, all the assorted items known in the trade as 'sundries'. Then he'd make his calls at small shops, enjoying the chitchat with shop-owners: in fact, the daily discourse was arguably more important than the business that was conducted. Taxes and traffic, crime rates, jokes, scathing comments about the city's football teams, Celtic and Rangers, lamentations on the Scottish weather, always the weather, *bloody cauld for the time o' year, intit? Ye'd freeze yer balls off in this*. And there were always the nomadic tribes of homeless alcoholics to talk about, the sad dispossessed groups that inhabited plots of wasteland between the tenements and lit fires to warm themselves when they couldn't afford to buy the cocktail that provided the heat they needed – usually milk spiked with hair lacquer. This was Sydney's Glasgow.

In the middle of the 1990s he's still doing the same job – he can never retire because that would deprive him of social contact with people who have almost become an extended family to him – but the Gorbals have been flattened by the wrecking-ball and its tenements replaced by new 'low-density' housing. Most of the inhabitants of the old Gorbals have been scattered to housing estates on the edges of the city, a diaspora regretted by many, because the relocation of thousands destroyed a valuable social entity – a community with roots, friendships and an entanglement of loyalties. Many of the wholesalers have been dispersed too, which makes Sydney's job all the harder. Now he has to travel sometimes to new warehouses in suburbs such as Rutherglen or to places, like Coatbridge, that lie beyond the city limits.

Sydney knows about the family skeleton, the sojourn in Scarborough, the whole charade that took place in 1955. He knows a child was born and given up for adoption. He has kept this shuttered in his mind for more than forty years. Even his closest friends, who have always suspected there was more to Doris's 'nervous breakdown' in 1955 than they were told, have never learned the truth from Sydney. He's protecting his sister. He's also guarding the dead. Honour thy father and mother. Sydney believes in what he's done – boxing this history down and nailing it shut and nobody's going to get at it. It's stuck away in the past; and the past is dead. So he thinks.

On the night of 2 August 1997, a Saturday – twelve days after I have come back from America, days of constant health bulletins and messages of hope and emanations of dread from Phoenix – the telephone rings in Sydney's flat.

A woman's voice: 'Mr Altman? Mr Sydney Altman?'

Sydney says it is.

'I'm trying to trace your sister. Eileen Altman.'

Sydney asks, 'Who am I speaking to?'

The woman has a Yorkshire accent. She hesitates a moment, then she replies, 'I'm Barbara.'

'Barbara?' Sydney can't place the name. Who does he know called Barbara? And then he remembers, and he thinks *no, surely not, this has to be some other Barbara. This can't be the child from all those years ago.*

But it is. The woman says quietly, 'I'm Eileen's daughter. I want to contact her. It's important. It's very important. I've been looking and looking for a long long time. I need your help, if you're willing, and I need it quickly . . .'

Sydney doesn't know what to say. His thoughts rush at once to the fact that Eileen is fighting for her life: what would a shock so seismic as the reappearance of a daughter she gave away for adoption more than forty years ago do to her position, already precarious? He decides to put Barbara off, stall her. 'This is a bad time. I don't know how she could handle the

# Part Two

# 13

A stack of letters and documents that came into my possession in the late spring of 1998 lies on my desk. Some of the letters are handwritten on blue-ruled paper with a ballpoint pen, others are flimsy carbons of office correspondence composed on a manual typewriter with irregular character alignments. For the most part the letters are dated between March and July 1955, but the earliest one was written on 26 June 1953 and sent to the York Adoption Society, from an address some thirty miles away in Harrogate.

*Dear Sir or Madam,*
   *My husband and I would like to apply to adopt a child.*
*We have been married 13 yrs & have no children of*
*our own. It is 7 years since we lost a baby at birth, & we*
*have had no sign of any more, much to our regret. So we*
*have decided we would like to apply for adoption.*
*If you would like to interview us, we are available to come*

*to York from the 11th of July to the 18th, as that week is my*
*husband's holidays. Hoping to hear from you.*

*Yours Sincerely*
*Mrs R A Wilson*

The handwriting is unadorned, the paper modest. You don't need clairvoyance to sense the sincerity in the letter. Seven years had passed since the death of Alice Wilson's infant, and there had been 'no sign' of another pregnancy; you can imagine the disappointments that had accrued in the thirteen years of the childless union between Alice and her husband Bob, a printer – summarised in that touching understatement 'much to our regret'. You can also imagine the consequences of the untimely death of a baby they'd obviously wanted desperately – the moments of depression followed by little flare-ups of fresh hope, conversations with their local GP, perhaps a consultation with a specialist, Alice's frustrations at failing to become pregnant, Bob's despair of ever being a father. As a last resort, they turned to the idea of adoption.

They awaited a response from the York Adoption Society. They worried if they'd be accepted, if they'd pass whatever tests were required of applicants before their names could be entered on a waiting list of prospective parents. Adoption societies were fastidiously careful, they didn't just go around giving babies away to anyone who asked – and the Wilsons wondered apprehensively, but with no good reason, if they'd fail to fulfil the criteria and never get a child.

In time, they were sent an application form, which they completed and returned on 4 September; three months had already passed since their original letter of inquiry. Alice was becoming impatient. Although she was a mild-mannered person in everyday matters, she was a bulldog when it came to the possibility of adoption. In an undated letter which must have been sent soon after they'd returned the forms, she wrote (clearly not for the first time) to Mrs Oloman, Secretary of the York Adoption Society:

> . . . *just a few lines from Harrogate again. Sorry to keep bothering you but I wondered if we were any nearer to getting on the list? I do hope so, as we are both getting older. Hoping to hear from you* . . . .

*Just a few lines again . . . Sorry to keep bothering you . . . we are both getting older.* Pressure of a gentle sort, but pressure just the same. Mrs Oloman, a patient woman obviously sympathetic to the Wilsons, checked the references they had provided – one from a minister, the other from a family friend – and found them to be in order. On 14 September 1953 she despatched Mr Gomersall, a children's officer associated with the Adoption Society, to inspect the Wilsons' home in Harrogate. It was a well-maintained terrace house in a working-class neighbourhood. Gomersall's report (missing from my file of documents, presumably lost or mislaid over the years) was submitted to Mrs Oloman on 20 October, and was clearly favourable, because the Wilsons were accepted and placed on the waiting list. Their stated preference was for a baby girl.

They might have imagined it wouldn't be long before they'd have a child, a notion quickly dispelled when Mrs Oloman wrote to explain the regrettable fact that there were more than thirty names before the Wilsons on the list. *Thirty unwanted babies to be found before Bob and Alice would get a chance!* That could take years. Forever. They might be too old when their opportunity arose.

Alice, with that determination of which Yorkshire people

are so proud, wanted to make sure her name was never far from Mrs Oloman's mind. On 10 December she wrote to Mrs Oloman:

> . . . *thank you for informing us about the waiting list.*
>
> *You mentioned that we had been placed on the list for a little boy, although on the forms we filled in we asked for a girl. Mind you, either would be welcome, but if we can have a preference a girl would be our choice . . .*

A girl would be 'preferred' to a boy; but 'either' would be welcome. The sex of the infant was of no relevance in the end. All that mattered was a child to fulfil the marriage. Alice was increasingly conscious of time rushing away from her and her husband; they'd first approached the Society in June 1953, and in January 1955 Mrs Oloman wrote to inform them that there were *still* twenty names ahead of theirs, and that 'very few baby girls were offered for adoption'.

Alice and Bob must have experienced fretful periods, impatience, and perhaps a sense of the unfairness of things – here they were, two decent people unable to have a family and all they wanted was to welcome an unwanted baby into the centre of their lives, and it just wasn't happening. I imagine Alice Wilson alone in the terraced house while Bob was at work, perhaps walking up and down the small boxroom she'd planned to turn into a nursery, and wondering how this phantom child would feel when – or if – she finally held it in her arms.

But the Wilsons found fortitude somewhere. In the only photograph of Bob and Alice I've seen, they have the appearance of people possessed of a quiet inner strength, a quality that stemmed more from their partnership than their individuality – Alice with her black hair and strong smile and summery 1950s frock, Bob in glasses and baggy flannels and sandals, his expression good-natured and trustworthy. He had the look of a man whose word you'd accept without question.

By April 1955 they'd managed to reach the relatively exalted position of number eighteen on the list – and how this sanctified list must have dominated their thoughts and plans and dreams! How they must have wondered if they'd ever reach the coveted number one position, as if it were some kind of popularity competition.

Their luck was about to turn unexpectedly. They received a letter from the Society dated 23 July 1955, more than two years after their first inquiry:

*Dear Mr and Mrs Wilson,*

*Due to a series of circumstances it has come to your turn for a baby rather sooner than we expected and we would like to interest you in a baby girl born on the 30th May, 1955.*

*Baby's mother is a single young girl, only seventeen years of age now. She's auburn-haired and of slim build, an exceedingly nice type of girl of whom references speak well. Her parents, too, are extremely nice people, who have helped their daughter in every way. It is felt she is too young to bring up this baby and better for the baby to have the love and care of both a 'Mummy and a Daddy.'*

*The mother is Jewish by birth but does not mind her baby being brought up in the Church of England faith. She has called the baby Barbara . . . We feel sure the baby will appeal to you.*

Mrs Oloman's letter also states that Barbara weighed 8lb 3oz at birth, that she was *a sweet little girl, fair at present and with blue eyes. The hair has perhaps a touch of gold in it.* (For a bureaucrat, Mrs Oloman had a nice eye for tiny colourful snippets.) The letter continues:

> *The mother and her parents wish to leave Scarborough by the end of July, so baby's adoption is rather urgent. We should like you both to come to this office and see Baby Barbara on Wednesday the 27th July, 1955, and if you liked her you would be able to take her home with you.*

To say that this news delighted the Wilsons would be an understatement, and in their high excitement they may not have paid too much attention to a sinister detail Mrs Oloman mentioned:

> *The mother was the victim of assault. She was attacked by a gang of young men, and this baby is the result of the incident. Not very much is known of the baby's father except that he was one of this set of young men . . .*

This is perhaps what Mrs Oloman referred to when she used the phrase 'due to a series of circumstances it has come to your turn for a baby sooner than expected'. But Mrs Oloman's information bore no relation to the story Eileen told me years ago when we went camping. No mention of a lover, the mysterious Bill. No clandestine love affair. No grand passion of the heart.

Officially, Baby Barbara was the consequence of a rape.

This version of events conveyed by Mrs Oloman to the Wilsons was based on information supplied by a certain Dr Caley, of Scarborough, who wrote to Mrs Oloman on 16 March 1955: *Eileen was the victim of an assault by a gang of hooligans in September 1954, as a result of which she became pregnant. She is in a depressed condition as a result of her*

*experience and pregnancy. I feel it would be the best for her if the
baby could be adopted as soon as possible after delivery . . . She
does not know the father as she was assaulted by three boys, and
they were all strangers to her.*

The official version. The party line. A gang of hooligans.
And where did Dr Caley get his information? Only from
Doris, of course. In a letter of 23 March 1955 to Mrs Oloman
on general matters pertaining to the adoption, Doris had writ-
ten: *With reference to the father of the child, I would refer you to
Dr Caley, who has all the information.*

As a way of protecting her daughter, Doris had already
uprooted herself and her family from home – so what was
another strand of fabrication to her at this stage? She'd shown
no curiosity about the baby's father; if she had questions of
Eileen, apparently she'd never asked them. Why not invent a
rape? In the hospital ward Eileen might have a soldier husband
stationed in Germany – it sounded romantic, separation from
a loved one performing his patriotic duty – but this fictional
spouse wouldn't convince Dr Caley, who'd have questions
about the soldier and the state of the marriage and the reason
for seeking adoption. So Dr Caley knew only what Doris chose
to tell him.

The Wilsons brought with them to York items Mrs
Oloman suggested in a letter – a shawl and a small case for the
baby's things. The Society provided some clothing, a bottle, a
tin of baby food, feeding instructions, milk books and vitamin
tokens. In a note attached to the file, written by an unnamed
functionary, the following is recorded:

*27 July 1955. Mr and Mrs Wilson came and saw Barbara
and decided to take her home. Baby handed over by Eileen in
front of her mother and Mrs Oloman to Mrs Davies of the
Children's Office.*

*Mrs Davies handed baby over to Mrs Wilson before Mrs Oloman.*

Flat unemotional language. The baby is 'handed over', the protocols of the transfer are observed by Mrs Oloman and Mrs Davies. Eileen didn't see the Wilsons. The baby was taken to another room. No mention of Eileen's tears. No reference to the joy of the Wilsons. The baby is moved from mother Number One to mother Number Two.

Eileen and her parents returned to Glasgow by bus, a long haul in the days before motorways. The Wilsons took Barbara home. They were predictably overjoyed with the infant. Within a matter of weeks they were writing to Mrs Oloman to tell her so; they included photographs of the baby. Mrs Oloman, whom I imagine as a good-hearted woman doing a difficult job she found immensely satisfying when she matched babies with parents, and who had to deal with heartache and disappointment daily, replied on 12 September 1955, to say she was pleased to receive the pictures.

*Barbara has certainly developed wonderfully under your care. No wonder you don't want to part with her. We have kept the laughing one and hope you don't mind. We certainly will not let Baby's mother see the photograph, so do not worry. She didn't say she wanted a photograph of her baby (often mothers do).*

Mrs Oloman was already in possession of a PRIVATE & CONFIDENTIAL report submitted to her by an Adoptions Officer called Joan Terton:

*The Wilsons are thrilled and delighted with the baby. Mr Wilson appears to take his full share of caring for the baby*

*and enjoys doing so. Judging by the spick and span appear-*
*ance of the house, Mrs Wilson appears to have adapted her*
*daily household routine most successfully. There is no doubt*
*that this baby has already taken her place as a member of*
*the family . . .*

Mrs Oloman had every reason to be happy with a job well
done; and so, at long last, did the Wilsons. As for Eileen, she
was left with the consolation of a thoughtful note from Mrs
Oloman, sent to her in Glasgow:

*Dear Eileen,*
    *We have heard today from Baby's adopting parents to say*
*how well she has settled in her new home . . . Baby has been*
*awaited a long time in this household and she has been*
*greatly admired by all who have seen her. She is a beautiful*
*baby. We are asked to tell you that she has completed what*
*was already a very happy marriage. I thought you would*
*like to have this news of her.*

I wonder if, when she read this letter, Eileen felt relief, or if
a tide of sadness overwhelmed her. *Have a good life*, she'd
whispered before giving up the child. And Alice and Bob
Wilson were exactly the kind of people to make sure that Baby
Barbara had as good a life as they could provide.

Barbara was immediately the focus of attention in the Wilson
household, and all her childhood memories were pleasant
ones. The attentions of Bob, the loving care of Alice, the big
attic room where she could bring friends to play as soon as she
was old enough to have any, the pet dogs she was allowed to
keep. She grew up, as she phrased it herself, 'in complete happiness. They were great parents.'

The question of what to tell Barbara about her adoption was something the Wilsons discussed between themselves at length. It wasn't an issue they were prepared to ignore. Seeking advice, Alice wrote to Mrs Oloman in February 1959:

*Barbara is nearly 4 years old and we are very happy with her. My husband and I are wondering what to tell her about her mother. Is it best to tell her that her parents are dead or to tell the truth? My husband thinks it's best to say they are dead, but we also don't like to lie to her . . .*

Mrs Oloman responded a few days later:

*We would not advise you to tell Barbara her parents are dead, but just stress that her Mother was very young and had her living to earn and so had to give up Barbara, and as you have given her all your love, I think she will accept the fact of her adoption as just part of her life with you.*

It was sensible advice, and the Wilsons took it. Barbara was told something about her real mother, but in such a manner that she couldn't have been disturbed by it. The sordid 'details' were omitted. *You were such a special little girl,* Alice Wilson said, *that you needed to have two mothers. You were chosen from a whole bunch of babies because you had the most beautiful smile.* For a time, this amount of information was enough – if you were five or six years old you could absorb it and get on with life in a world you were just trying to make some sense of.

But the tiny seed sown in Barbara's mind would sprout, and put forth questions as addictive as any narcotic leaf. Who was her birth mother? And where was she? Despite the childhood she called perfect, Barbara found herself wishing, as she grew older, that she could let her 'real' mother know she was in good care, that she was loved. This frustrated longing was always at its most powerful on her birthdays, when she woke with what she called 'a lonely sadness and yearning for her mother'. (And Eileen – did she feel an emptiness on 30 May each year? If she did, she never said as much to me. And I detected nothing. But did she carry the weight inside her? Was there a small passing dull ache? I never knew.)

So Barbara was already living in two spheres – the tangible one that immediately surrounded her, with all its easy familiarities of parents and friends and toys, and the other where there were profound mysteries to be solved about her origins, and a mother whose voice she had no memory of ever hearing, and whose face she couldn't imagine. The compelling biological curiosity, the fundamental *need* to know who you are and where you came from, was beginning to resonate inside her, sometimes so quietly she could live with it, but often with a persistence she couldn't ignore.

In 1967 Bob Wilson was diagnosed as having cancer of the liver. He was briefly hospitalised – his condition was beyond surgery – and he was sent home to die. Barbara, twelve years of age, read to him and fed him small amounts of food, sharing responsibility with her mother during her father's last few weeks of life. On the morning of Bob Wilson's death, he was laid out on his bed with a clean white handkerchief spread across his face – in the customary fashion of the place and time. Barbara remembered being alone with the body, and lifting the corner of the handkerchief to look at her father one last time: saddened, she found him 'peaceful but yellow'.

Bob's death reinforced Barbara's desire to find out more about her biological mother. Whether it was because she felt insecure, whether life seemed suddenly a very delicate edifice to her for the first time and death a blind brute force, she

asked Alice how to go about locating information. Despite
her own grief and stress, Alice was helpful. Maybe she saw the
same determination in her daughter she'd seen in herself when
she'd first set out on the long road to adoption. Barbara
wanted to know more about her 'natural' mother, and *nothing*
would stop her.

Alice contacted Social Services, who furnished a minimum
amount of information. Mother's name and age at time of
birth. Religion. Nationality. And the address of the house
Doris and Issy had rented in Scarborough. That was all. But
Alice felt obliged to raise the circumstances surrounding
Barbara's birth – the 'true story', which couldn't have been
easy to tell after more than twelve years of holding it back.
How to inform the child you love of this wretched fact: *you
were the product of violence. The accidental outcome of a forced
communion of strangers.*

Alice told the story as it had been relayed to her in Mrs
Oloman's correspondence, and it affected Barbara intensely; it
was a story she'd believe for a long time. Through all the years
of searching that lay ahead of her, she believed she was the
offspring of rape. A knife, a scream, a penetration in the dark,
a hand locked across a wet mouth: was it like that?

She later wrote: *It truly did not matter to me, I just wanted to
find her. I remember when I heard people say things like 'you've
got your mother's eyes' I used to feel a kind of loneliness, a quiet
sadness . . .*

*A quiet sadness.* I walk around the house under an Irish spring
half-moon. The night's silence is undisturbed. It seems to
me, in a fanciful moment, to extend forever, all the way from
the heart of the bog to the rocky shorelines of this island and
then beyond, out across swollen oceans to those places that
are always named on maritime weather reports on BBC radio

in the depths of night. Mizen Head. Finisterre. Fastnet. Lundy.

I think of the handkerchief on Barbara's dead father's face and I associate it with a memory of my socialist grandfather's corpse laid out in a coffin in the bedroom of a tenement flat in the south of Glasgow not far from the river, and I am eight years of age, and my father asks me if I want to look at my grandpa's body, and I think *no, I don't, aw Dad, please don't ask me to look*, but I look anyway, standing on tiptoes and gazing over the rim of the upraised coffin and seeing my grandfather, white and dead and very small, dressed in a shroud the colour of buttermilk. I'd never seen a dead man before, and I'd never forgotten that lifeless face – the *emptiness* of it – and now it comes back to me in the eerie silvery quiet of the Irish countryside.

The phrase *a quiet sadness* plays inside my head again. If Barbara began her search in childish earnest in the late 1960s when she was only twelve, then by the time she was old enough to pursue it with the resources of a young adult, Eileen was already three thousand miles away on an odyssey of her own – a fresh shot at our marriage, a new beginning in a new country.

# 14

WE arrived in Oswego in the early 1970s. An icy town located on the shores of Lake Ontario not far south of the Canadian line, a college community dominated by the sinister grid of the Niagara-Mohawk power plant, it had some fine leafy streets and elaborate turn-of-the-century homes; but it was generally rundown, bisected by weed-choked railroad lines along which decrepit freight-cars rattled. The shore, where dead fish poisoned by lake water rotted in their thousands, resembled a lifeless planet in a remote galaxy.

Oswego, I thought, might provide salvation – a new environment where our marriage would flourish, a place where we'd prove that we were still a going concern. I hadn't quit drinking after Stephen's birth the way I'd intended at the time; with the contrary logic of the drunk, I'd quit publishing instead. I'd gone into my office on Golden Square in Soho one April morning, sat behind my desk for a few minutes, smoked a cigarette, stared at the walls, the schedules, the artwork for assorted book jackets, and I was struck by the stifling pointlessness of it all. Book galleys, proofs, manuscripts, sales figures – what did any of this matter? The joy had seeped out of the business; what had begun in a love affair with language had become drudgery. With no consideration of consequence, no consultation with Eileen, I wrote a letter of resignation from Granada – a life-altering decision made on the sharp pinhead of a moment.

I'd published two novels by this time, written one TV play, a third novel had just been bought by the firm of William Collins; I had no idea what I was going to do other than write more fiction – which wasn't going to bring in enough money to pay the mortgage and the bills associated with two small sons, unless I were visited in the night by that fickle slut, the Fiction Fairy, who bestows riches on a few writers at random.

Without much hope of a favourable reply, I wrote to my former English professor at Sussex, David Daiches, about the possibility of an academic position somewhere. I liked Daiches, an intelligent Scotsman and excellent teacher, who also happened to be an expert on the subject of single malt whisky. He referred me to Baxter Hathaway, a professor of literature at Cornell, who wrote to say he'd heard of a position teaching creative writing at the State University of New York at Oswego. I'd never taught, never heard of Oswego; I sent a note to the chairman of the English Department, an affable Anglophile called Bill Drake, who telephoned me within a few days of the receipt of my letter and offered me the position. I accepted. (I later learned that he'd acted on the 'psychic' advice of his wife, a powerful woman given to melodrama, who'd 'sensed' an indefinable quality she seemingly found acceptable in my letter. Hire this man, she'd told Bill, holding my letter to her forehead and catching God only knows what 'emanations'. Later, I'd come to wonder if the heavy-duty wires reaching out from the Niagara-Mohawk power plant emitted waves that interfered with normal brain activity, mine included.)

Neither Eileen nor myself had been in the USA before. But what the hell. Go for it. Make the break. We located the town on a map. Nowhere, USA. (The only place of any size in the vicinity that sounded familiar was Syracuse.) Oswego, we read in a guidebook, had a population of around 15,000, which included about 5–6,000 students. The teaching schedule offered to me wasn't demanding – six hours a week; the salary, tax-free for a year, was good compared to publishing.

A year away from London – liniment for the soul. I'd convinced myself that our frail marriage could be shored up, made good again, if only I could quit drinking, be responsible, pull myself back from that brink where drinkers go in their nightmares, those high wires where they strut in defiance of gravity – but this could *only* happen if I escaped the snares and lures of London, and Soho in particular. The drunk's dictum: always blame the place, not the person. I sometimes wondered what it would be like not to drink, to be one of those people who called themselves teetotallers, but the concept of abstinence was a step too far.

We left London late at night, two adults and two small baffled innocent boys, four refugees, to catch a cut-rate charter flight to JFK from Heathrow; Eileen wept sadly in the car before we'd even reached the end of the street, she wasn't sure about this huge step, she'd come to enjoy living in the suburbs of London with kids and garden, she was more settled than I'd ever realised. I felt clumsy at having uprooted her so thoughtlessly. Why hadn't I discussed it fully with her beforehand? Because I was in a hurry – me me me, watch me move, get out of my way – I didn't want to slow down and weigh the good

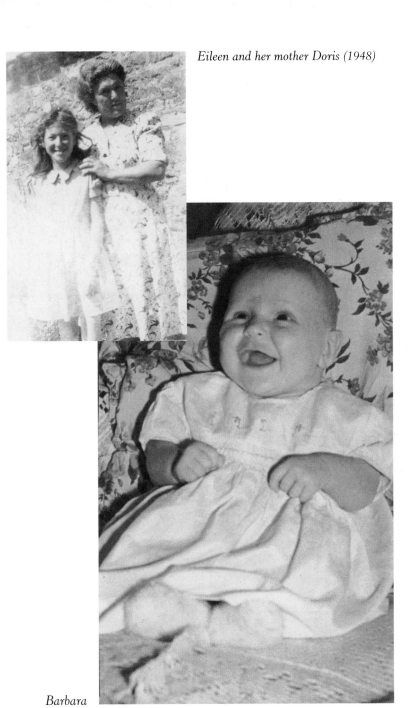

*Eileen and her mother Doris (1948)*

*Barbara*

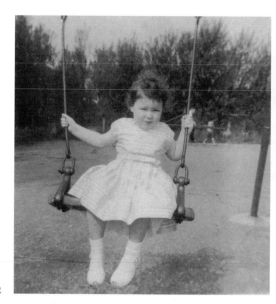

*Barbara*

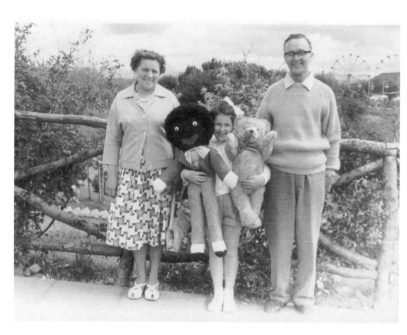

*Barbara and her adoptive parents, Alice and Bill*

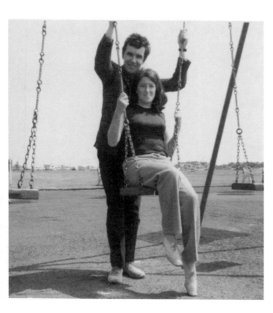

*Campbell and Eileen,*
*Broughty Ferry, (1969)*

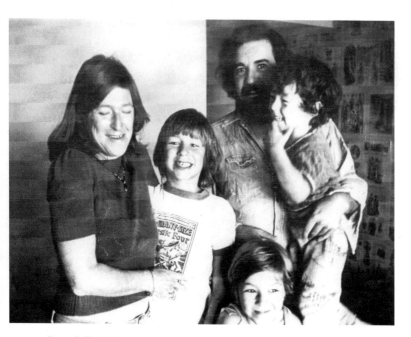

*Campbell, Eileen, Iain, Stephen and Keiron, Arizona, (1976)*

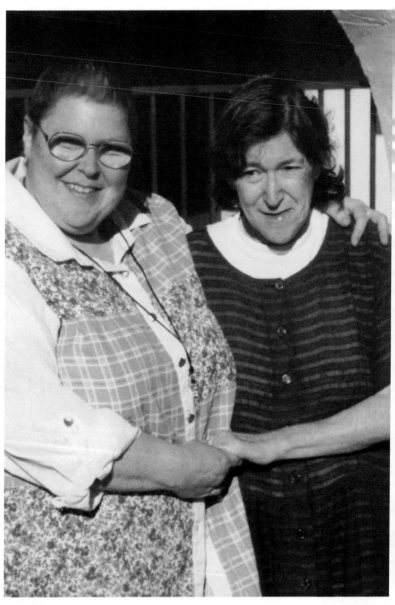

*Barbara and Eileen, shortly before Eileen's death (Christmas 1997)*

and the bad, I didn't have mental or moral scales calibrated so
finely as to make an accurate measurement of the two in any
event, I *lunged* towards America without due thought, I was
scared of staying in London and wrecking myself, and I
dragged Eileen and the kids in my jet stream all the way to
upstate New York.

She knew why I felt we had to go. The marriage had hair-
line fractures – but did we have to fly so goddamn far to apply
the splints? She wanted to know why we couldn't solve our
problems without having to dash three thousand miles
through space. It was a terrific question and, like all terrific
questions, it had only one answer: *we didn't have to make the
trip at all*. You move your problem to another country and the
only thing you adjust is your wristwatch to a new time zone.
Your heart's chronometer doesn't alter.

Eileen knew more about psychological baggage than me,
and she understood you couldn't jettison it halfway across the
Atlantic, you carried your luggage with you and declared its
contents at every port of entry on your life's itinerary. And all
the time I was thinking: *dammit, I'll make this marriage work,
I'll be a different man, I'll be a good man and a good husband, I
only need a fresh start elsewhere*. I'd felt the same sense of
unlimited possibilities the night of Stephen's birth, the notion
I could soar if only I knew how to be free of my puzzling self-
destructive twinges. So: Oswego (an easy anagram of So We
Go: was that a good omen?) was the promised land with the
odd name. This is where I'd become worthy, dependable, the
iron spine of my small family. But what I sensed in Eileen's
misgivings was the simple proposition I chose not to acknowledge: you don't escape from your self.

I had no preconceptions about the place, I wasn't expecting
or desiring high culture, stimulating intellectual life; I was in
the market for a change of scenery, a quiet corner of the

world, a frame house with a porch like the kind I'd seen in
American movies and TV shows. I imagined being a true
Daddy. I imagined ballparks and hot dogs and my kids speaking American and having to utter the Pledge of Allegiance
every morning at school. And a flag fluttering in the background, red and white and blue – the colours of liberty – in a
country where it was always early Fall, the landscape gently
changing.

All my images of smalltown America had been force-fed
me through the filter system of Hollywood, and they were
false and hypocritical and sanitised, as they had to be. The
America we entered was a country simmering with post-
Vietnam unease, troubled by racial tensions, lorded over by a
President who'd treated the constitution like toilet paper, and
was looking into the shotgun of impeachment. It was a land
stretched on a rack of self-doubt. Patriotism was an ugly word.
There were no war heroes coming home to smalltown ticker-
tape welcomes and decent jobs or easy business loans, a quick
handshake with the friendly bank manager, a wink, *Well done
in 'Nam, Joe, anything you need, boy, you ask, the country owes
you bigtime*. This was no I Love Lucy dreamtime, no George
Burns talking to his TV audience over a Dutch door in a
make-believe town called Beverly Hills. As a backdrop against
which to fix the faults in our marriage, America wasn't exactly
a model of stability.

The country seemed to me to be located at an intersection
where Babel met Bedlam. There was chaos about. Rumours
were running loose in the landscape. People claimed to hear
subterranean voices planning conspiracies. Furtive think-tanks
were said to be buried under the Rockies manipulating the
world money supply. Corporate America lied to the good cit-
izens about the safety of certain pharmaceutical drugs and
tobacco, and big munitions deals were conducted in paranoid

secrecy, and the DEA, gearing up for the so-called war on drugs that Reagan and Bush would later find such a vote-basket, sprayed the marijuana fields of Mexico with the poison paraquat and torched the cocaine labs of Colombia, and sinister persons allegedly attached to obscure government research departments freely passed out dangerous experimental narcotics to America's waifs in the Haight-Ashbury and other clapped-out places where freewheeling kiddie dopers gathered and collapsed. When Richard Nixon fired Archibald Cox, the Special Investigator into the Watergate burglary, somebody hung a banner outside a campus building in Oswego with the legend: *Nixon Is A Coxsacker.*

It was a nation going mad. Nobody knew the rules, and the book of regulations had been lost. It was crazy time, all bets were off, the politicians had shafted the populace, tens of thousands of young boys were dead in a bullshit war, mantel-pieces and coffee-tables in homes throughout the country had framed photographs of sons who were never coming back from the jungles and paddy fields of hell, there was a great groundswell of heartbreak, and the Commander in Chief was borderline psycho – so let's party, why not?

Morality? That was a word in a foreign tongue.

Ominously for me, Oswego had more bars to the square mile than anywhere else in Christendom and because it snowed for five or six months of the year social activity was usually limited to the corner tavern. On blizzardy nights with visibility at a few feet, you couldn't get very far anyhow. Snow was the main topic of conversation everywhere. Lyon might be proud of its silk, say, or San Francisco its sourdough bread, but Oswegonians were wondrously pleased with their *snowfall*. They talked excitedly in the bars of legendary blizzards of the past; they told macabre tales of cars that had been buried for months on end, people locked solid in stationary vehicles and found, frigid and pinched, at the first thaw. They took great delight in the legends of past winters. People died out there. They blundered around in blizzards and sometimes a few had been known to slip off the bridge into the roaring Oswego River and that was the end of them. When old-timers talked of a twelve-foot overnight snowfall, they had the bright-lit eyes of gold prospectors drooling over tales of fabulous lost mines.

Snow isolated the town, gave it a sense of unreality, as if it were not attached to the rest of America but had broken loose. Fierce blizzards blew off the lake and roared across the campus with such strength that hapless pedestrians were obliged to hang on to a safety-rope for fear of being picked up and blown downstate to the Finger Lakes like so many matchstick figures.

We'd settled into a house on the east side of Oswego. Eileen seemed comfortable in this little corner of America, where British-style formalities were almost nonexistent, and she became friendly with some of the other faculty wives, many of whom went out of their way to make her welcome. I taught my classes. I didn't have a clue what was expected of me. I mumbled about dialogue and character development and the use of detail; I had the distinct feeling that at any given time only two or three students out of twenty had any interest in the subject – and these were usually young women who sat near the front of the room in their bell-bottoms and see-through peasant blouses with beads hanging from their wrists and throats, and who often found a reason to linger after class asking inane questions.

I was, I knew, something of a minor curiosity in this place – I had a Scottish accent not much modified during the years since I'd left Glasgow, I'd published novels (this had an inexplicable appeal for some people, even a mild glamour), I wasn't any kind of faculty establishment figure, a standard-issue visiting Brit professor with leather patches on the elbows of my tweed jacket and a pipe and a pontifical look, I was young, wore my hair long, dressed casually. I was accessible during office hours, and if anyone missed me then, I could always be found in one bar or another, if you knew where to look – and in a small town it was never hard to locate anyone. And I didn't take the work with professorial seriousness. How could you *teach* another human being to write fiction? You could *edit* someone's work, sure, but that was the limit of what you could genuinely contribute. Any other claims were hogwash.

The marriage went along well for a time, although Oswego wasn't a place for easy redemption; for one thing, I was still drinking, although in a slightly less frenetic way than I'd done in London. At least initially. (Trying to be good, trying *hard* to be *good*.) For another, grass was freely available, and so was LSD. Marijuana wasn't my narcotic of choice, it didn't have the kick of booze that made you want to be gregarious, it was all a little too introspective and caused me to brood, but I smoked it regularly anyway.

Eileen smoked it with me from time to time – I think she saw it as a kind of marital bonding; if her husband was going to use the drug, she'd keep up with him. Something in common. An experience shared. It often had freaky effects on her. Once, she refused to come down a short flight of stairs because some invisible, indefinable terror lurked between the top step and the bottom, and although she could 'see' it she couldn't describe it. Grass made her outrageously adventurous at times; one wintry night, she insisted on making the forty-mile trip through a raging blizzard to Syracuse because she was obsessing on Chinese food, had to have it, couldn't live without spare ribs – a dope fixation she herself found hilarious. She drove off into the snow with a friend of ours, and came back with a paper sack of cold Chinese food, some of which she'd devoured on the return trip. Her fingers were sticky from plum sauce, and her smile as impish as that of a child who'd secretly eaten the last of the Christmas pudding.

I drifted into The Affair without thought: I could claim that. I could say I was seduced, and I wouldn't have trouble believing that judgment. I could say that alcohol played a major role in the indiscretion; and that too would be true up to a point. But these are excuses. The truth is simple and raw and I can't tuck it under layers of obfuscation. I wanted the woman, she wanted me; we were on a hot collision course from the first time we met. She made the first move; young American women were more sexually aggressive than their British counterparts. They stalked and they hunted and they did so without any subterfuge. You could all but see the invisible bow in the hand and the quiver of arrows slung across the shoulder. K, a student, long-haired and mahogany-eyed and earthy and single-minded, belonged in this category.

An infidelity. Some men let the word roll off their tongue even as it rolls out of their memories. Nudge-nudge, a bit on the side. A meaningless little dalliance. Nothing to get worked up about, buddy. I couldn't deal with it that easily; some inherent Calvinist trait made me feel bad, low, heartsick, but booze numbed regret and applied a little anaesthetic to self-contempt. I'd betrayed my wife, the woman I'd hauled all the way across the world – and for what? So that I could commit an act of treachery? Bring her anguish? Hide behind lies? Where was this fresh fucking start I'd wanted to give her? I might have shoved the whole matter inside that drainpipe where memories you don't want are stuffed; I might have walked away from K – but it didn't work out like that, because I wanted to see the girl again, and she me, and so began a regular relationship of some intensity.

The context offered an appropriate setting; the drug culture was the background against which people lived loose lives, a fact that created a kind of soft cushion for me against *total* self-loathing – my behaviour wasn't *that* extraordinary, my actions weren't *that* terrible, were they? In this small campus town people were changing partners with the frequency of participants at a square dance. It was commonplace. I wasn't the first married man to stray (there's a sweet euphemism), I wasn't going to be the last, so why I was making such a big deal out of it, it happened, life wasn't all faithfulness and happy marriages—

But these were just feeble straws and provided no support for what I was doing, which was going to hurt Eileen; and she didn't deserve that. I wanted to break off the relationship with K. I don't remember now how Eileen found out about it, whether I told her in an inebriated confessional moment, if she heard stories on the smalltown telegraph, if gossip buzzed, if she guessed instinctively, if I left clues that were easily found (this is the most likely, a few giveaways) – these recollections are lost, bleached from my head.

She said in that remarkably quiet way she sometimes had – deliberating over each word, choosing to say precisely what she meant, staying calm, keeping her emotions in check – that she needed to think about the situation, what she was going to do, how she was going to deal with it. Dear Christ, I thought, she was a long long way from home and I'd brought her more pain. Was I ever going to grow up and realise that relationships needed gentle nurture and attention and unselfish care if they were to thrive?

I moved out of the house for a time. I avoided K, didn't answer her phone calls. I didn't telephone Eileen either to ask how she was coping, how the boys were reacting. She'd developed by this time some close friendships with a couple of faculty wives, whose marriages were also troubled; there was a mutual support system, I knew; feminism was on the rise too.

I went into a kind of zombie withdrawal. I was in freefall. Alcohol and a very strong strain of grass rumoured to be the legendary mind-wasting Rangoon Red – these were my maintenance systems.

I remember living in a room over a liquor store. A mattress on a floor, and blinds drawn. A room in somebody's apartment where I stayed for a while. Mice rustling over old newspapers in the night. I remember a prolonged stupor and disconnected images of my wife and sons and K, and I thought how rancid everything had become, we should never have come to America in the first place, *stooooopid* idea, and the mice cavorted among the papers and built nests and gave birth and I didn't open the blinds and every so often somebody in another room would fetch alcohol or food, obliging spectres coming and going in my perpetual twilight.

When I finally went out I took absent-minded drives away from the squalor of my room into the countryside. There was an austere wintry beauty about this part of the world when the sky was brilliant and cloudless, the ground thick with snow, the tall pines blackly mystifying. A lonesome sort of loveliness. Frozen water reflecting a cold sun, a solitary hawk in flight – this landscape filled me with indefinable longings, even a slight little touch of apprehension. I had a sense that what you saw was only the picturesque outer rim of the place, that if you went any deeper into the forests you'd encounter ravenous animals and the ferocious savagery of nature and blood on the snow.

Eileen came to see me in my room one day. She said nothing about the revolting shabbiness of the place.

*The boys miss you,* she said.

I said I missed them. I asked, *What have you told them?*

*Just that you needed some time to yourself. They want you to come home now.*

She'd protected the kids from a hard truth. Daddy's gone. He has another woman. She'd spared me and I was grateful.

I asked her what *she* wanted.

*I want you to come home too,* she said.

I told her I wasn't seeing K any more.

She said she knew that. She'd heard. She touched my hand. *We have to give this a try. We can't give up on it now.*

She was opening a door for me. She was inviting me back inside, where it was warm and safe. I hated this room above the liquor store. I despised the drift of my life, and my ruinous appetites. I missed her, and I longed to be with my sons.

*Let's forget all this crap,* she said. *Come home.*

I didn't hesitate. I stuffed my belongings in a brown paper sack. Mice rustled in the trash in the fireplace, building their homes out of cigarette butts, crumpled Tareyton cigarette packs, food wrappers, old newspapers. Eileen listened to the sounds with a puzzled look.

*Company,* I told her.

My contract at Oswego was extended year by year to a total of four. Four blinding white winters and four swamplike summers, days of killer humidity. We bought a house for $13,500. The place had dubious foundations, the surveyor said. Was he talking symbolically? We liked the house. A third son, Keiron, was born in Oswego Hospital, our American child. Eileen found a job working with children at the campus day-care centre; it was the first rung on the ladder of a future she couldn't have imagined at the time.

I spent some time refraining from alcohol, a dry interlude. It didn't last. I'd known it couldn't. I had a malicious bug in my system that was constantly thirsty. I loved Eileen, and her patience, and the ability she'd developed to transcend my times of wild behaviour. But the drift was beginning again, for her and for me, and the warmth of our reconciliation was escaping like hot air through a flawed radiator valve. She floated into a brief affair – which took me by surprise, and caused a pain quite unfamiliar to me, a spasm in the heart, a great falling, I deserved it, but what was I supposed to say?

She had every right. She had been given the licence to do it. God knows, I'd stamped the document myself. Inevitably, I also embarked on the steamship Infidelity again. Names elude me now, faces and bodies vanish in firelight or candleflame. Memory is like a kind of alphabet soup where too many vowels are missing for you to reconstruct whole words, you only get fragments. Girls came and went and the ship kept sailing. Who remembers it all now?

Everything was coming apart. We were committing manslaughter on our marriage. Unless we wanted to break up entirely, we had to move elsewhere. Move again. Keep moving until you get it right. Blame the place, always *always* blame the place. And so, after four years in Oswego, we found ourselves heading to Arizona. Our first attempt at a new life hadn't worked out; maybe we deluded ourselves into thinking that, in a vastly different climate, we'd perform a more lasting act of restoration.

I'd been offered a teaching position at Arizona State University, which might have been situated on the other side

of an unknown moon for all I cared. I pretended I wanted it;
I deceived myself into thinking – yet again, dear God, what a
master of self-delusion I'd become – that westward lay
redemption. Something certainly lay to the faraway west, but
it wasn't redemption.

I remember the long road trip from upstate New York to
Arizona, the three kids in the car, the family dog – a benign
English setter; I remember the monotony of the highway and
the impossible chore of occupying the time of three small
restless kids on a 3,000-mile drive – colouring-books and
crayons and paper games; motels on the edge of freeways,
chlorinated pools where the kids could release their energies,
smuggling the dog into rooms where no animals were allowed.

Any photograph taken of us during that trip would have
depicted husband and wife and three little boys, faces in the
sunlight, smiles – like any family heading towards a new life in
a place where grapefruits and oranges grew on trees and the
sun shone all the livelong day: a paradise.

# 15

WHEN Alice Wilson died of a heart attack in 1979, Barbara's loss was immeasurable; she was involved in the ongoing search for Eileen, but Alice was the only mother she'd ever known. She was married by the time of Alice's death, and four months pregnant with her first child, and although she was happy with her life and looking forward to the birth of her baby, she was still very much perplexed by the unanswered questions about her biological mother. Who was this teenage girl who'd given birth to her? What was she like? Where had she disappeared and what had become of her? How to solve the mystery? Barbara had made a few exploratory probes over the years, but she'd always run into a bureaucratic cul-de-sac, as if the destiny of her mother were a secret too great to divulge. *We can't tell you anything. That kind of information is confidential.*

She'd innocently entered an intricate maze whose only path to the exit on the other side was presided over by clerks and functionaries and social workers, men and women who kept truth stuck in locked filing cabinets and password-protected computer disks. Truth was their personal domain; they could

dole it out in dribs and drabs, or they could refuse to admit its
existence. When Barbara contacted Social Services personnel,
which she did many times, she was always told the same
thing – she could gain no further access to information beyond
what she already had, her mother's name. On one occasion, she
was even informed that the building where adoption records
were stored had burned down, a monstrous item of bureaucratic 'misinformation' worthy of a Stalinist apparatchik.

She understood that this was the system's way of protecting
Eileen's identity, given the 'official' circumstances of Barbara's
conception. But she wasn't to be deterred by policy or those
who implemented it. She kept a journal about her search for
her mother: in one entry she wrote, *After each knock back, I
just get on with my life. I'm low and depressed for a while, then the
yearning comes around again and I seek out new support groups,
only to be told they can't help me. Each time I go to Social Services
offices, I'm interviewed by well-meaning but condescending social
workers. I go through the routine of having to convince them that
I'm sure I know what I'm doing by looking for my mother.*

She was tempted every so often to place ads in newspapers;
but she knew this wasn't the way to go about finding Eileen. If
Eileen had married without telling her husband about the
adopted baby, the consequences of a newspaper ad could be
embarrassing, disastrous.

At one point, Barbara wrote to a popular TV programme
called *Surprise Surprise* which, unashamedly sentimental,
reunited long-lost relatives, brothers and sisters who'd been
separated by family circumstance, or parted during wartime,
adoptees, old sweethearts who'd lost touch. It was Kleenex
TV. Barbara imagined that she might be one of the fortunate
ones chosen, and researchers would locate her mother and put
her on the show, and Barbara would get to meet her for the

first time under the bright lights of the studio – *surprise surprise!*

She heard nothing from the producers. She was optimistic enough to interpret this silence not as lack of interest – but as evidence that the show's researchers were exploring her story in depth, and they'd be in touch with her eventually with the news that they'd located her mother. It didn't happen. Even her letter of inquiry wasn't acknowledged. But she never gave up; that just wasn't in her personality. Each blind alley, each time she was overlooked or ignored or patronised, only strengthened her determination to continue. What she called 'the yearning' in her journal wasn't going to be silenced by rejection.

At times, her search was interrupted for long periods by family matters, or other issues that absorbed her. She became engrossed in the subject of dyslexia, because her own children (she had three by now) suffered from the affliction and, along with other parents, she began campaigning actively, lobbying members of the education authorities to give dyslexics special instruction in schools. She was passionate in pursuit of this goal, and eventually became 'parent representative' on the interviewing panel for prospective teachers; she played a sig-nificant part in raising the standards of instruction for dyslexics in local schools. Barbara fighting battles, waging wars, all flags flying and guns blazing – if she was persistent in the matter of Eileen, she was just as resolute when it came to whatever strong beliefs she held.

Even at the heart of her serious work on behalf of these kids, she dreamed up a little fantasy that concerned her mother. Was it not within the realms of possibility that one day some serious-minded talk-show producer might want to present a programme on the subject of dyslexia? And what if he or she were to ask Barbara to appear as a guest, because she was knowledgeable by now, and she had a position of some

influence locally? And maybe she'd walk inside the studio
where, by sheer chance, she'd just happen to run into the TV
personality Cilla Black, the star of *Surprise Surprise*, and she'd
engage Cilla in conversation, telling her about Eileen, and how
she'd written to the producers and never received a response,
and Cilla would be very nice and understanding and she'd
smile in her toothy trust-me way and pat Barbara's arm and
say, in her Scouser accent, *Of course we can help, love, no problem, we'll find your Mum, let's sit down and have a nice cuppa
tea and a long chat* . . .

Hope, sometimes so simple, can often become elaborate; an
accumulation of *what ifs,* like an unstable edifice of brightly-
coloured kiddie building blocks. Barbara's life was rich with
hope, and ripe with dreams. And sometimes those dreams were
not very grand at all, indeed they were often touchingly modest:
in the event that she located her mother, and Eileen didn't want
to see her, for example, Barbara had a back-up plan ready. She'd
watch her mother secretly, from a distance. She'd see her go in
and out of shops, or maybe she'd arrange to get her hair done in
the same beauty parlor at the same time as Eileen, and they'd
fall into casual conversation – and Eileen would never know the
woman in the next chair was her lost daughter. *If that is all I
can have of her,* Barbara wrote, *I'll settle for that.*

Sitting in a parked car and observing her mother walk past;
trailing her from a distance along a sidewalk – these tiny acts
of espionage wouldn't have satisfied her. She wanted what she
called 'blood-ties', the fundamental security that so many
other people take for granted.

*Blood-ties;* her fuel. It wasn't just a search for her mother
alone, although that was paramount, but for a wider family
network too – aunts, uncles, grandparents, cousins. She was
looking for answers to the big questions. Who was Barbara?
Where did she belong? Where had she really come from?

Sometimes she wondered why she couldn't just forget this quest and be content with the life she had – husband Nick, who loved her and had always encouraged her in the hunt for her mother, daughter Heidi, a pretty girl who worked in a residential nursing home, and was as much friend as a daughter, an intuitive, bright young woman; her two sons, Mat the fanatical football-player, the joker, the clown of the family, the kind of kid with the knack of raising people's spirits; and Marcus, the perfectionist, happy with mechanical things, stripping down bikes and rebuilding them. They were decent kids who adored their mother and needed her. A cheerful family, a comfortable home surrounded by the starkly dramatic, sometimes romantic landscape of the Yorkshire dales, am exuberant household filled with life and noise, the scent of tobacco from Nick's pipe and the budgerigar that hung upside down in its cage and wolf-whistled to attract the family dogs, the stout two-foot long gurami fish that could be fed bits of fruit by hand – wouldn't all this have been enough for most people?

Maybe. But it wasn't enough for Barbara. It never occurred to her to set aside the matter of Eileen; it was a constant in her life, this sense of an absence, an amputation. And so she contacted all kinds of support groups, adoption societies, national adoption registries, Salvation Army sources – always with no result. She registered with NORCAP, the National Organisation of Counselling for Adoptees and their Parents, but this was fruitless, because it depended on both mother and daughter registering their names, and so expressing a mutual desire to be reunited.

Eileen, six thousand miles away while Barbara was actively looking for her, had never expressed any such need, and she'd probably never heard of NORCAP anyway – and even if she had, she wouldn't have done anything about it. As she herself said some time later: *There was not much reason to hope I'd ever see Barbara again.* It was a notion so far-fetched it wasn't worth thinking about.

Besides, Eileen had other matters to deal with, three sons and a new job and an unpredictable husband and a marriage drying up under the wicked suns of the Saguaro desert, that landscape of the bleached bones of long-dead steers and the frail skeletons of cactus wrens picked clean by hawks and human corpses buried beneath red scrub by the Arizona Mafia – and Barbara was a whisper from another age, a name trapped in a room nobody ever entered.

It rains in Ireland as I write; one of those soft soothing rains behind which some hint of sun hangs. Irish rain, Arizona sun: extremes. A life of extremes. After the numbing winters and humid summers of Oswego, Phoenix was a dry corner of hell. We rented a house, I went off to teach creative writing again, the boys attended school, Eileen decided to look for work.

Arizona State University had all the charm of a series of large motels strung together to form a small city. It had a student population of around 40,000; it might have been designed with enforced loneliness and alienation in mind – the crush of student pedestrians hurrying anonymously between classes, the big faceless dormitory slabs, the pervasive impression that human contact was minimal in this place, it hadn't been planned for friendships. It was a conveyor belt environment. It wasn't education; it was forcing pork into a sausage-skin.

ASU was a jock college; academic standards were secondary to gladiatorial conquest. I got polite little postcards from coaches asking me to give passing grades to near-illiterates who just happened to be promising running-backs or who knew how to shoot baskets. As far as I could tell, the sports

teams gave the campus its only sense of unity or identity. I felt
no kinship with the place; it wasn't the screaming sunlight
that disaffected me, and it wasn't the jock attitude to education – it was my lack of interest in what I was doing with my
life: *teaching*? Why was I still *teaching*, for Christ's sake? What
was the point of ploughing through these handwritten character sketches and short exercises in dialogue that students
turned in? Where was it all supposed to lead? I hadn't written
anything in years, and sometimes I was beset by panic – *I'll
never write again*. I was all burned out. I'd risen briefly a little
way, then fallen to earth.

It was easier to walk from the campus across Apache
Boulevard to a small old-fashioned bar called Frank's Friendly
Tavern than to wrestle these dogged, muscular problems.
Frank's, operated by a whining sabre-rattling old misanthrope
who never moved more than a few inches from the cash register, appealed to me hugely. Rundown, patronised by barstool
cowboys, trailer-park denizens, bikers, an occasional doper
student, it was a temple of beery worship and refuge from the
tribulations of the cosmos – and also from the miserable
understanding that the marriage wasn't working any better
here than in Oswego. We'd come all this way with great hope,
*false* hope, and now . . . What next? Would I soon be asking
Eileen and the boys to uproot and move with me another three
thousand miles, an academic post in Mexico City, say, or
teaching English in Lima?

*Listen, Eileen, it's going to be better down there, I hear life is
sweet . . .* I imagined our lives as a series of journeys, staying in
ever more obscure outposts of the world for very short periods
of time. A year in Bogota, six months in La Paz, and on southward, as far as we could go. Sombreros and ponchos in
Patagonia. Rearing sheep or goats in an unforgiving landscape.
The kids speaking Spanish. The end of the world. Running,

running, performing quick fixes as we went. Stephen would write later that his mother was the anchor of the family; 'Dad was always busy trying to get us settled wherever we were, and that was usually someplace different, always on the move.'

Always on the move. Yes. Always. I couldn't keep still. I was a fugitive from myself, my devils. Alone, this might have been of no consequence. But I had a wife and kids, and I drew them along in my wake, and I gave them no say in the matter. I'd hauled them from Brighton to London to upstate New York and now to Arizona. This pattern of restlessness raised too many questions whose answers eluded me: was I trying to impose on real life the design I could force on fiction? Did I want the people in the world to be like the people in my books? Was it deeper than that – did I even *know* where reality ended and fiction began, or had that line of demarcation decayed long ago, without me ever noticing it? I wasn't sure I wanted an answer to that question; or if I did, could I find one?

Eileen wouldn't want to move, even if I raised the preposterous possibility again. She'd found a job working with handicapped children in South Phoenix at a place called the Hacienda. She'd discovered, to her own surprise, that she was good at this work. It excited her. It was different from the day-care centre in Oswego, she was challenged by the kids, who were often hopelessly retarded. She had the patience to cope with them, devise diversions for them, win their confidence; in a short time she was promoted to programme supervisor. She didn't have the academic qualifications normally required for this kind of job, but she had heart in abundance, and willingness and dedication, and she was smart.

The position restored much of the self-confidence our marriage had eroded. She was a capable person, she had something to offer the world, she wasn't just a housewife who hated the drudgery of being housebound and seeing the stack of dirty dishes in the sink, and the grubby fingerprints of little kids on the door panels and walls; she wasn't just another woman with a husband who drank too much, she wasn't somebody who stood in her spouse's overbearing shadow, she could be more than that, far more – and I was proud of her too, I was pleased for her, because the Hacienda fulfilled her in ways I couldn't.

It would be false to claim I was drinking out of frustration. Or I was drinking because I wasn't happy teaching, depressed that the books weren't flowing out of me like spring water. The truth is different: I was drinking because I still *liked* it. No: *I loved it*. The buzz, the high, the unpredictability. My mood had no connection with my drinking. Up, down, happy, sad, there was no relationship between my state of mind and my alcoholic intake. Excuses? I didn't need them. Nor, astonishingly, did I think for a moment that alcohol was a *problem* in my life. After all, I could go a week or ten days without drinking, without even thinking about booze. If it was really a problem, wouldn't I be drinking *every* day? Hell, I still had control. I could drink when I liked.

As for hangovers – they were a little more demonic, more enduring, than they'd been before. But they never lasted for long, half a day at worst. Dehydration, shakiness – these were inconveniences. Sometimes a little cocaine, which I'd begun to use now and again, would magic the hangover out of existence entirely. Whip through the sinuses, clear the head, give the sleepy nerve-endings a brisk wake-up call. Dunk the cobwebbed brain in a shower of sparkly white powder.

And then there was the new phenomenon that had begun to occur on hungover mornings, the one I called The Faces. The Faces would form somewhere at the back of your head and they were always vaguely familiar, like composites of people you knew in real life, but as they floated closer they changed, they morphed into heads more reptilian than human, some horned, others scaly, others distorted beyond any easy category of recognition: my own horror show. But a problem? No way. The Faces would vanish as soon as you opened your eyes.

The children – of course, they noticed my drinking. How could they fail to? I was often late for dinner, sometimes I didn't show until they were fast asleep and I'd tiptoe into the house, blundering through the dark. I convinced myself they understood me, sympathised with me, perhaps found me amusing in an eccentric way. But it was their mother they turned to more frequently for friendship than me; it was with her they shared their confidences. They could tell her things they couldn't tell me. Many years later Iain wrote that his Mom was his best friend, someone who was there when his father was absent.

One afternoon, motivated by the need to play the Good Father, to make amends for some recent oversight or disappointment I'd inflicted on them – I forget what: there were so many – I bundled Stephen and Keiron, aged ten and eight, into the car. (It was a beat '68 Chevy Malibu that had survived assorted skirmishes with unexpected physical obstacles, although the lid of the trunk was weirdly crumpled from an incident when I'd backed into the wall of a dive called Six East in Tempe. Why was I drawn to these pits?)

I drove the kids to a sleazy fair in the shadowy no man's land between Tempe and Phoenix, a shabby midway long since demolished. Let them have some fun, an outing on a sunny day, let them shoot air rifles at clay ducks or ride the bumper cars or whatever they wanted. I wandered around. The place, which had a bad reputation and a dodgy clientele, was crowded. The sky was high and blue and the sun was hot. I was thirsty. The kids had wandered away. I walked until I found a bar. I needed a drink. The heat, the sun. I was sweating. One drink, two, three. I sat in air-conditioned heaven. Four, five, six. Time melted as it always did in bars. Circuit-breakers in the brain sizzled and shorted. The kids. I knew they'd be fine. I'd go round them up and take them home in another . . . oh, fifteen minutes. Seven, eight drinks. Time to go. Outside, it was late afternoon and the sun was falling. How long had I been in that bar? I figured an hour. But it had to be more. Two or three. Four maybe? I didn't have a watch. I looked through the crowds for the kids, couldn't find them, I pushed against the flow of people, I checked the arcades, the stalls, the rides, the alleys behind the stalls, those places where thick tangles of electrical cables lay here and there carrying ominous currents, I couldn't find the boys, I was stumbling through a white sunlit nightmare looking for two lost kids, through air that stank of hot dogs and beef burning and onions, where were those boys? Had they been abducted? Had they been stolen from me? O Jesus Christ. How could I find them? Where was I supposed to look? The flow of people kept coming, I collided with this person, that, I bounced through the throng with strident panic roaring inside me, *where were my goddamn children?* Pennies rolled down chutes and tinny music crackled from cheap sound systems and a Ferris wheel turned in the clear air, but there was no sign of my sons, and I loved them so, and if I'd lost them forever – the noisy fears and anxieties that tumbled through my mind were amplified by the loudspeakers of alcohol.

I telephoned Eileen: what to say? I mislaid the kids? I can't find them? They've vanished into that place of dread where lost children go and are never seen again even though you search the face of the planet all your life, following half-assed clues and unconvincing sightings?

She had a sharp edge of anger in her voice. 'You abandoned the kids and they called me and I picked them up.'

Relief, relief. Thank you, God. I'd go down on my knees. 'I didn't abandon them exactly,' I said.

'What would you call it?'

I didn't have an answer for that. I didn't have a word.

'You've been drinking,' she said. She always knew. Even if I'd had only one drink, a *sniff* of a drink, somehow she knew from my voice.

'I had a couple—'

'We need to talk, Campbell. We can't go on like this.'

After I hung up I thought: she was right. *We couldn't go on like this.* No life, except for the most self-destructive, could be conducted this way. She wanted to make serious changes; she was convinced things could get better. And now, in one of those turnabouts that mark subtle shifts in relationships, it was she who was reassuring me. We have to work at it, she said. It isn't going to be easy. But it's worth it, to rescue our family. Think of what we've gone through together, all the ups and downs, the partings and reconciliations. Think of the boys.

What she proposed was family counselling. She chose the counsellor, arranged the appointments. I remember how much faith she put in these sessions, how hard she tried to hold our family together, how eager she was to cooperate with the counsellor – a dark-haired tough-minded pretty woman who stood about four-feet nine inches. It was a sombre time, a trying time, as if Eileen were attempting single-handed to salvage a ship that had sunk some years ago. I helped so little. At times I felt like a voyeur listening to the innermost secrets of a broken marriage that had nothing to do with me. And the boys, who attended some of these sessions, often seemed embarrassed, or became awkwardly silent; they wished their family life was normal, that it wasn't a drama played out in front of a fierce little counsellor who asked hard questions.

Eileen worked on in her own brave way. This was the sad part, this is what hurts me now as I remember – she was flying solo, and I don't think she knew it, she thought I was sitting alongside her in the cockpit; I could hear a note of dangerous uncertainty in the drone of the engine, and Eileen was going to come flaming down out of her flight path. I wanted to help her fly this goddamn kite. I wanted to participate, be her co-pilot. I wanted to make this family strong and whole again. I wanted. I wanted.

But I couldn't help, I couldn't find it in myself to come out and say what I'd slowly come to recognise as an irrefutable fact: I didn't love her the way she wanted. I didn't love her the way I'd done once. I didn't love her in a way that made the perpetuation of family life possible. I saw a marriage held in place by the adhesive of kids and the tentacles of habits, and I was aware that these arrangements frequently collapsed in misery and recrimination. I'd changed, the structure of my love had altered; and Eileen, if she'd been totally candid with herself, if she'd funnelled her energies into accepting truth instead of counselling, might have come to the same conclusion – or so, rightly or wrongly, I believe now.

She'd changed too. She'd discovered the possibilities of a new career. She was suddenly independent, she was feeling stronger, better about herself. She was a new person, but she was still trying to cling to the structures of an old life. And it couldn't be done. Maybe she was still afraid of the new. Maybe her confidence hadn't blossomed entirely at the time.

Whatever the truth, she was steel-willed in her determination to make the marriage work, and apart from the counselling sessions she also arranged for me to see a psychiatrist, who spoke to me for about half an hour on the effects of drink, and then prescribed Librium, nineteen caps in all, an odd number – take two the first day, two the second, two the third, and then reduce to one a day until the medication is gone. And then what? I asked.

*And then I don't want to see you again*, he said.

Why not?

*You're verbally too skilled.*

I was never sure what this meant, or why the shrink would find a communicative patient a threat. It didn't matter. I didn't want a close encounter with myself, or to be analysed, or to be put in touch with my hidden feelings.

By this time in my life I'd met Rebecca.

*Bzzzz, bzzzz gggggrrrrrrzzzzzzzz* – I can hear from my office the sound of a man slicing through the hard wood of a storm-felled tree with a chainsaw, and the air is clear and sunny after the recent rains, and rooks distressed by the harshness of the saw flap fearfully away across fields. I perform the morning ritual of pricking my fingertip for a drop of blood that I can place on a chemically treated strip of plastic I insert into a device, a glucometer that measures the sugar in my blood. The read-out in the little window is seven point one, quite acceptable. I wonder sometimes if all the years of drinking contributed to this diabetes. My physician tells me no. I don't draw any conclusions from this – except that diabetes might have been punishment for the long years of self-inflicted abuse. I should be beyond all this now, this idea of punishment for deeds done and hurts imposed; but sometimes the old urge to nail yourself to the crooked scaffold of your history is strong.

I think of Eileen and our marriage and how it all drew finally to a close. But the sound of the saw outside keeps intruding on my memories – grating, filling the air with chips of wood and fine dust. Maybe this is an appropriate sound anyway, because it conveys something of the teeth-grinding quality of the end of the marriage, the rasp-throated sadness of parting.

Rebecca was a graduate teaching assistant in the English Department at Arizona State. She was small and slim and moved in a graceful weightless way; she'd been trained as a ballet dancer. I liked the elegant structure of her cheekbones and how her long brown hair fell to her shoulders. I liked her intelligence and her feisty quality. But there was no immediate leap into a relationship. She was writing a novel and I was reading it, making comments and suggestions, and that was as far as it went for a long time. I enjoyed her company, we had writing as a common interest. Now and then we'd have a drink together, discuss books. I asked her to edit a novelisation I'd been commissioned to write for the comic-book film *Raiders of the Lost Ark*. She had a good sharp eye for editorial work.

Sometimes months would pass between our meetings. The relationship was friendly, and hadn't gone beyond that. Inevitably, though, it did, it combusted – and it happened just as Eileen was still hoping that the counselling sessions would result in conjugal miracles.

And – I fell in love. This was no casual affair, no quick spin on the old sexual roulette wheel: this was Big-Time, this was the carousel trip when the heart expands, and your pulse beats a little harder than it has done in a long time, and your thoughts border on obsession, you can't get a name and a face out of your mind. The world becomes electric. You're shocked, and all your senses jangle. I'd tried to avoid Rebecca, and she me – Christ, how we'd tried – but these attempts at evasion were pointless, and we both knew it.

I wanted to walk away from the relationship. I wanted to be able to scream with huge enthusiasm – yes yes yes Eileen! Let's put our lives in the hands of the counsellor! Let's do it!

Let's keep on the straight and narrow! Don't stray again. It leads only to chaos. Play by the rules you agreed to years before in a register office in North London, Campbell. Yes yes Jesus yes! I was scared of hurting her. But the pretence was too great, the part too difficult to act out with any conviction. How do you tell your wife that you love somebody else? That although you've tried to avoid this encounter with another love, and ignore it, make it go away, that you've stood in call-boxes and dialled half the digits of the other woman's number and then hung up because you knew where the completed call would lead, how do you tell your wife that this feeling keeps returning, zoning in on you, scudding into your dreams uninvited? How do you tell her you've been blitzed and the ground is opening into fissures under your feet? How do you tell her these things? How do you say, look, this woman makes me happy in a way I haven't felt in years, our marriage is over now, how in God's name do you utter such statements and keep any hold on dignity and decency, and escape the straitjacket of guilt?

We spoke together hesitantly about the situation, Eileen and I. She was sad that I was unhappy. She was sad that our marriage was a lost cause. I told her I'd stay with her, that by some stretch of will we'd make it through, we'd look back on all this one day and shake our heads in disbelief – but this offer wasn't one she was willing to accept. And how could she anyway, knowing I'd carry an absence in my heart, that there would be a winter between us always?

And that was when she went to see Rebecca. That was when she told Rebecca I was going to be unhappy if I stayed inside the marriage. That perhaps Rebecca understood me in a way that she, Eileen, had never managed to achieve. And in that moment Eileen decided to step out of the picture. That was the day she told me: *I just gave you away* – and she stuck her hands into the pockets of her jeans and looked past me, as if she were trying to make out something in the distance, or in the future, and her eyes were wet. I wanted to reach for her and say *We can't let this happen, we'll wake out of this night-mare, remember all the good times we had, the old Glasgow days, the Brighton days, the trip we took to Philadelphia, the time we got stuck in the snow on a trip to Montreal and the car broke and it would only travel in reverse gear, remember the humid vacations in Virginia Beach when the kids were small, the drive to Kitty Hawk and Cape Hatteras and the wooden houses on stilts, and the visit to Williamsburg, remember remember, o love, let me take you away from all this pain,* but my words would have been unconvincing.

*I just gave you away.*

Dear Eileen, who never knowingly hurt anyone. Stephen told me years later that after the final break-up he'd sit with her far into the night when she was depressed and smoking cigarettes continually and sometimes she'd hyperventilate. He said, 'Nothing else in the world mattered to me but the happiness of my Mum. I wasn't mad at my Dad, because I believe Mom wasn't mad at him either, it was just that she was trying to get used to the process of changes taking place.'

As Eileen had given Barbara away long ago, she now gave me away. She deserved better than to make sacrifices for the well-being of other people. Far better.

With Rebecca and Leda and Keiron, a new family, I headed north in the mid-1980s to Sedona, a place whose extravagantly awesome sandstone scenery seemingly affected the minds of the town's inhabitants, turning their thoughts to a variety of New Age matters – some of them utterly weirdass, concerning UFOs and planetary convergences and vacationing aliens who borrowed human bodies for walking around in. Jeeps painted bright pink would rattle you through allegedly 'positive vortices' in the landscape, if that was what you wanted (I didn't); there were people prepared to convince you that great benefits might be had from hanging crystals in your window (I remained steadfastly sceptical). It was a town of spiritual sleight-of-hand artists, fortune-tellers, tea-leaf readers, palmists, odd religions, false gurus, fake healers and sad self-deluded seekers, many of them fugitives from California hunting The Big Truth they hadn't been able to discover in the canyons of Los Angeles.

The Big Truth. I wondered if I'd come to the right place. All I wanted was peace in which to write, and a good truthful relationship with Rebecca. And sobriety; yes, Lord, sobriety.

Ignorant of the flux of her mother's life, uncertain even of her existence, Barbara visited the Register Office in Leeds to search for a copy of her mother's birth certificate. But she found none – which meant that Eileen hadn't been born in England, Wales or Northern Ireland, otherwise the fact would have been recorded, the document duly filed. Another dead end.

She continued her quest when she could, when the needs of a busy family life didn't intervene. But she was running out of options and ideas. She couldn't afford a private detective to look. She still didn't want to advertise. How would she phrase such an item anyway: *Daughter Seeks Long-lost Mother*? And where would it be printed, in *Lost & Found*? In *Personal* – among requests for dates and friendships and all the lonely voices crying out to be heard?

So where else could she go to find evidence of her mother's life and whereabouts? There was one place she hadn't tried: Scotland.

# 16

In the autumn of 1996, before she could plan her trip to Scotland, Barbara became sick. Extreme menstrual pain, sweats, excessive fatigue; her first reaction was that these might be symptoms of menopause, although she was only forty years old. She had a blood test performed to measure her hormone levels, which were normal. She wasn't menopausal. She was examined by her GP, and then referred to a gynaecologist who gave her an ultrasound scan; it revealed cysts in both ovaries and fibrous tissue in the uterus. A 'routine' hysterectomy was scheduled to remove the cysts. The uterus couldn't be saved. The operation went well; the procedure was commonplace, after all.

Four days later, as she waited in her hospital bed expecting to be discharged, the nurse came into the ward and, without explanation, closed the privacy curtain around the bed. A few minutes later, the curtain parted and a tall grey-bearded man stepped into the cocoon. He was a consultant. Barbara knew instantly that whatever he was going to say would be serious.

He had a brisk manner and wore gold-rimmed spectacles and a bow-tie.

Despite her feeling of foreboding, Barbara tried to remain calm. 'You're going to tell me something I don't want to hear. Right?'

The consultant was the kind of man who came straight to the point. He didn't know any other way. He'd spent his lifetime relaying medical information – good, bad, indifferent, it didn't matter which – to his patients. 'The lab telephoned to say that the cysts in your ovaries were in the first stage of cancer. You're one very lucky lady – if you hadn't come in for the routine op, you would have been dead within two years. The next step is to zap you with chemotherapy. I'm not absolutely sure you need it, because I'm satisfied that the surgery worked, but if you were my wife I'd give you chemo as an insurance policy.'

One very lucky lady? Cancer? Zap with what – *chemotherapy*? Wait a minute, hold on, stop the clock: this was surely some mistake. Later, Barbara would recall the eerie atmosphere in the tiny curtained space, how silent everything fell, how the stripes on the consultant's suit seemed to become more vivid; but most of all, she'd remember how fear had paralysed her.

In his matter-of-fact manner, the consultant said, 'We'll start you off with six treatments, one a month. The drug we'll be giving you won't make your hair fall out, so you don't have to worry about that.'

*Baldness!* That was the least of her concerns. She was terrified; her life was collapsing all around her. She could hear the walls of her world being ripped out of the ground and blown away. She was in the middle of a tornado, and unprotected. What did hair loss matter, for God's sake? She felt she'd been transported suddenly into hell. She'd boarded a dark-lit boneshaker old bus whose journey was strictly one-way; there was no round-trip available on this run. She felt physically altered, as if somebody had set fire to her scalp and shoved sharp needles into her face. Her private landscape was cracking and hissing underfoot.

Cancer, Jesus Christ – what was she supposed to tell her husband and kids? Cancer, the dark unmerciful vampire, blood-sucking, leeching off veins, had walked into their own back yard. How did you break the news to other people that you were living under a shadow of death when you couldn't absorb it yourself? Was she just to be seized away from everything she knew and loved by this treachery inside her own body?

Barbara made an understandable decision; she wouldn't tell her husband Nick at once. Whenever she had to go to hospital, she created little stories, dental appointments, a visit to an optician, anything that suited her purpose. She kept it all to herself. It was seven weeks and two chemo treatments before she found the courage to confide in him: he didn't panic as she'd halfway expected – instead, he was surprisingly calm and provided the support she needed. And she needed it all the more when, during her fourth treatment as an outpatient at the hospital in March 1997, her tumour marker test, which had been in the acceptable range of about ten, jumped to sixty-nine.

*Sixty-nine!*

She lost control, she was panicked and scared and all at once everything was chaotic and she started shouting, '*How can that be? How can that possibly be? How can it be sixty-nine? Oh God. Oh God!*' She was rushing here and there around the consulting room, raging and waving her arms and screaming before she was ushered into an office to be calmed down. The consultant was called in, and all Barbara could think of was how she wasn't getting better, her situation was deteriorating, the treatment wasn't working, she was going to die. There was talk of more blood tests, more scans, oncologists coming to examine her. Chemotherapy was suspended while she waited for a new scan to be arranged and an appointment made with cancer specialists.

From her nursing experience, she knew cancer's voracious appetite, and how, like rust, it was never still; it grew until it was beyond control. She began to develop a cough and a tightness in her chest and complained of shortness of breath. By the time she went for the new scan, which was restricted to her abdomen and diaphragm, she was coughing hard. The picture showed a suspicious lesion on the large intestine, and a small nodule on the diaphragm.

The lungs, though, lay outside the scope of the scan.

Now other specialists became involved, and on 30 May 1997 – her forty-second birthday – she had a meeting with them. The results were bad, as she'd known instinctively they'd be: there was cancer in her colon. She was given chemotherapy in the form of the drug Taxol, which meant she'd lose her hair within three weeks of treatment. Was it only a few months ago her world had been reasonably normal? What had happened to the healthy Barbara? She'd vanished under an avalanche of sickness; her life had become a bad news bulletin. And there was worse to come.

She was increasingly short of breath, coughing more and more. She knew there was something seriously wrong inside her chest. She asked for an X-ray. It was with a feeling of dread – now a constant companion, a cloaked figure following her around like a malevolent shadow – that she learned the result: cancer had metastasised in both lungs and had spread to the chest glands along the diaphragm, as well as some of the lymph glands. The cancer had not only spread, it had taken up occupancy in sites of Barbara's body that were inoperable. It was a family of evil tenants who couldn't be evicted, murderous squatters who couldn't be excised with a surgical knife; a family of killers, assassins inside her, in her cells.

In June 1997 she wrote in her journal: *I am looking into the face of death. I must find my mother immediately.*

This old Irish house is allegedly haunted. Doug, the former owner, an amiable Canadian told me this as I signed the legal papers. 'There's a presence in that house, laddie,' was how he put it. One story you can hear in local pubs involves the devil's face appearing in an upstairs window that has subsequently been blocked off; another concerns a priest who committed suicide for some reason. Rebecca has had experiences here of a supernatural nature, and so has Leda; other guests report strange dreams or feelings. I've had only one unusual encounter, when a benign presence, unmistakably female, tucked in the side of my bed-sheet, and I felt a soft careful movement of a hand, a passage of air gently, warmly, stirred. It may have been nothing more than the product of my half-sleeping state, but I want to think otherwise. What kind of barren prosaic world is it without spirits? I was alone in the house at the time, so I can't ascribe the event to any human agent. When I looked around the bedroom, I saw nobody, heard nothing. The presence – whatever it was – had vanished.

What is undeniably true is that the site of the house has seen considerable violence and destruction down the centuries – in the 1600s Cromwell, the Great Arsonist, burned a castle here, people were killed, cannons fired, and in the 1920s members of the old Irish Republican Army were hidden in an upstairs room by the family that owned the house. Much of the history of the place is lost, unrecorded, distorted and enriched by centuries of oral tradition. But the notion that the house is haunted lingers on. Sometimes, looking the length of one of the corridors, I'm struck by how shadows collect in the vaunted ceiling, how they gather between the great curved ribs of plasterwork.

If ghosts come and go along these corridors they do so quietly, the way images float through memories – the way Sedona, Arizona, comes back to me, in a series of shifting pictures, impressions, no hard black-and-white edges, shimmering recollections of the old wooden house Rebecca and I bought on the edge of the National Forest, some five miles out of town; we had it stripped down to its skeleton and remodelled. For a time we were happy in this dry red dusty place twenty miles south of Flagstaff. Rebecca opened a studio and taught ballet. Keiron and Leda went to local schools. And I wrote. I had a couple of successful novels and a lucrative contract for another few books.

I was in touch with Eileen from time to time; we talked about Keiron and how he was doing in school or we discussed her new job at a clinic in downtown Phoenix. Although the clinic was chronically underfunded and salaries often paid late, the job – caring for seriously brain-damaged children – excited and engrossed her. These kids, near-drowning victims, survivors of accidents, the congenitally retarded, came to Phoenix from all over the world. Eileen had received training in the treatment known as 'patterning', which requires extraordinary patience; it's repetitive and demanding and often downright grinding work.

I didn't ask about her personal life: I had no rights in that matter. I knew that after our separation she'd been seeing a man called Michael, and that for a short time between jobs of her own she'd helped him at his work trimming palm trees. (I have a distinct memory of seeing her one burning hot Phoenix day in T-shirt, denim cut-offs, blue and white head scarf, carrying a long scythe-like tool used to lop fronds from palms, sweat running down her face to her neck.) Michael, who had marital problems of his own, eventually drifted out of the picture. I understood, from the passing references she made, that the relationship was at times turbulent and disturbing. (Later, there were other men, although these relationships don't seem to have caught fire. Peter, a married man with a severe case of Catholic guilt, apparently preferred steamy phone calls and letters to real encounters: a 'virtual' romance that Eileen wanted to transmute into something more real, but it went nowhere. And Richard, another with no future; also a married man, he'd leave gifts inside her car or notes on her windshield, but he drew back when it seemed to him that his wife was becoming suspicious.)

At the close of our conversation, Eileen volunteered the fact that she was beginning to take an interest in dreams, and dream analysis. I had the feeling she was moving in directions I couldn't follow, or maybe I didn't want to; maybe it was just a little too strange for me at that point in my life.

Rebecca was urging me to deal with my drinking; I hadn't stopped, and didn't seem able to make that break. I disappointed her time and again as I'd done to Eileen – arrangements overlooked or forgotten, erratic behaviour, rampant unreliability: was my life to be the same plot of land spaded over and over until the day they buried me in it? One hungover morning, my hand heeby-jeebying, I telephoned Alcoholics Anonymous, and somebody was despatched, like a roadside mechanic sent to make a repair *in situ*, to bring me to a meeting. He was a small fey man, a professional fortune-teller, which in Sedona wasn't an uncommon occupation.

I felt uneasy at the AA meeting; it was such a volatile mix of hope and fear, depression and cheerfulness, smugness and insecurity, that I didn't think I'd be able to straighten myself out in a room so clogged with assorted emotions. I also didn't like the religious aspect of AA, the Higher Power concept (I'd been playing around with a half-assed atheism for years), nor the way in which some people with years of sobriety assumed a kind of spiritual aura, as if sobriety alone licensed them to be Grade-A gurus and empowered them to grasp a hidden inner level of meaning in *The Big Book*, AA's Bible. There was also much hugging and weeping, and self-congratulatory sobriety birthdays – *I've been sober for six months! Awright! Far out!* – and sad tales, many of them variants on one theme: self-destruction. I realised that there was nothing unique in being a drunk. *So I drank my life away. Lost my goddamn job. Wife and kids upped and split. Haven't seen or heard of 'em since. I tried suicide, see these scars on my wrists? Spent years in therapy. Went to residential clinics. Stayed sober a week then got drunk for the next seven years. Got a job as an engineer onna railroad and drove a hunnerd ton of coal dead drunk across Louisiana one night and don't remember a goddamn thing about it. And here I am at this meeting tonight, sober for thirty days. Thanks, guys! Thanks for being here when I needed you! And if I slip I know you'll still be here.*

The Slip. Oh, the dreaded Slip. Avoid at all costs. You may have been sober twenty years, but the Slip was just around a corner, waiting like a hired gun.

I began to attend daily meetings. I went to ones that started at seven AM because I liked the small number of people in this group; and I loved the air at that time of morning, especially on sunny wintry days, the fir trees black-green, the formation of mysterious shadows in the clefts of red rocks, the sky a blue of such purity it stalled your heart.

I quit drinking for several years. It wasn't as difficult as I'd imagined, I didn't find myself longing for booze the way I'd expected. I had uneasy moments, little white-knuckle drum-rolling cliffhanger episodes – drink, don't drink, will he, won't he, in the great scheme of things who gives a damn anyway – but these receded. Sometimes on a book tour, if I was far away from home, I pondered a beer: who'd know anyway? *Me. I'd know.* So I didn't give in. I had layers of uncharted resolve, the discovery of which pleased and surprised me.

Drink was duly vanquished – what next in the abstinence stakes? I quit smoking. Oh, sainthood was within my grasp. I could smell the cleaning fluid on my halo. Lead me to water and I would have walked on it. I wrote books, earned money, kept appointments, became *dependable*. Rebecca could rely on me. The kids began to have confidence in me. I felt at ease in the world. I drove past bars where I'd formerly drunk, my brain like a busted gyroscope, until closing time; in my sobriety, I even fished drunks out of bars on a couple of occasions. If you're going to be Clean & Sober you go the whole way, or you don't go at all. This was the new me; I developed the bold swagger of a man who can conquer all his bad appetites.

And then the demons inside, who'd only been dormant when I'd fooled myself into thinking they'd been *exterminated*, woke up, chattering like maddened red-eyed primates. Cunning little fanged bastards, they sensed it was feeding time. They'd been deprived too long and they were ravenous and they rushed in their grunting, hump-backed way to feast on me. *Get that booze down your gullet, my man. And while you're at it, how about some dope?* It's wake-up time, slough off that cowl of respectability, which doesn't suit you.

I began the slide down; it was the easiest thing in the world. I didn't resist, didn't complain, didn't fight the monsters; I realised I'd been waiting for them all along. So I took up residence in the clammy tin-shack border shantytown of Slipsville, a slum world of hot flashes and linguistic

breakdowns and blackouts and a feeling of freon in the brain.
Narrow streets going nowhere and dim doorways and The
Faces watching you from rusty balconies overhead and the
sound of a pianola clunking out *The Honky-Tonk Blues* and air
stinking of stale booze and madness everywhere.

Nobody sleeps in Slipsville. The place has no motels, no
flophouses, no beds to rent. Who needs beds? You stay awake
all the time. You drink. You drink some more. You do cocaine
and it jangles you and your heart shudders, and again you
drink some more to smooth the tense manic edges of the drug
which has been cut with God knows what, the laxative
Manitol, bad bathtub crank, maybe Vitamin C if you're really
lucky. I wasn't swaggering sober-headed now. I was hardly
walking upright.

Slipsville is all crooked angles. Everything is skewed, doors
aslant, drawers don't close, shutters hang tilted from windows.
Slipsville is where you find yourself sitting in an alley in a
parked car while somebody you hardly know – just a fellow
traveller with the same demons gnawing on him, just some
guy you encountered in an end-of-the-world bar – goes off
into the dark in search of the magic connection. Slipsville is
where you find yourself walking beneath the palm-tree shadows of unfamiliar trailer parks at three AM looking for a fellow
you understand you can score from, and he's usually some
tattooed grunt with a vocabulary of about eleven words and a
Colt forty-five or a double-barrel shotgun and a set of scales
and glassine packets of white powder and a hardcore porn
video playing in his trailer and *you have to be pleasant to him,
you have to grovel to this baboon*. It's where there's no moon,
and no memory the next time you wake up.

And one night you return, bent out of shape, mind utterly
shot, to your house, and it's dark and empty. And so's your life.
In the vacant rooms you hear your wife's voice echo: *don't feed the*

*demons, Campbell. Don't feed them.* So you walk these rooms and you think: *what happened to me, I was a good person only a few weeks ago and now I'm alone and Rebecca's gone and so are the kids.*

Outside, there are shadows between the pine trees, and in your demolished mind these shadows get twisted around, and you know – beyond *all* doubt – they're not *shadows*, they're people moving on all fours towards the house. They have every intention of surrounding it. They're after you. In the room upstairs, you can hear footsteps. Somebody's up there too. Maybe more than one. They mean you harm. Switch on all the lights, inside and out, flood the place with light. See who's there. Hello. But there's nothing in the lights, only trees, maybe a raccoon moving, a skunk slinking past. You rush upstairs. Nobody's there. Check the attic. Nothing. This is sickness, madness, self-imposed. You chew the dry inside of your mouth or grit your teeth and even though you know there's nothing out there in the forest and nobody else in the house – all the same you can *still sense* presences about you, and they're malignant, they're horrors, mutants from the inner city of Slipsville, and they're coming after you. By jeep and bus, by foot or by Harley, by hook or by crook, by whatever means of transport they have, they've travelled here to get you. Because you're sick. Because you're hallucinating. Because you haven't slept in three nights, or is it four? You're being way-out-there irrational, but that doesn't stop these fuckers pouring in from Slipsville, some dressed in Cuban-style camouflage gear, others in cowboy shirts and jeans, and they're all armed; and now the house is surrounded by them, and you huddle up on the kitchen floor, knees raised to your face, and trembling you wait. *Hey Gringo! Hey dude!* We're coming in. Voices. Whose? Nobody is out there. Nobody. But I hear them shout and I hear them move. I need a downer, I know somewhere there's Valium, I've seen it . . . where, what drawer, what closet, what

cabinet, what bottle? Rummage, fumble, things go clattering to
the floor, but where is that Valium? Search the toothpaste tubes
and the soap and the drawers that contain combs and razor
blades and decongestants and assorted over-the-counter cold
remedies – no goddamn Valium. You dreamed it. Another figment. Like the Cubans. The cowboys. Like the feeling that
Exocet missiles or Scuds are being wheeled into firing position
in the night hills overlooking the house – all part of the same
nonstop insane nightmare.

I'm breathing bad and hard and my nerves are frazzled. I
stand at the glass doors that lead to the deck and I watch the
forest, and dark gives way to the first oystershell moment of
dawn. In daylight you're safe. When the sun rises you'll be
fine – but you won't be fine, not really. Because your head's
not straight and you feel like dying and the hangover is thick
in your throat and there's not a damn thing in the house to
drink and no drugs left. I move out on to the deck and my life,
I realise, has become a wasteland of causing pain to other
people, and imposing grief on those who've loved me. And I
need, God in heaven, an end to it.

Will somebody tell me when the next bus leaves Slipsville?
I want out of here badly, I want sleep, sobriety, clarity.
Normality. To be whole, to be well, even to be honourable –
*yes*, to gather the bits and pieces of my life and staple them
back together once and for all. I'd do it, godammit, somehow
I'd do it. I'd had a glimpse of that other person I could be
during my years of sobriety, and I wanted to be him again –
even if it meant moving yet another time to yet another place,
I'd get where I needed to be. Away from this lunacy, this land-
scape I've populated with phantoms. Somewhere new. Fresh.
Different. A continent away, a vast ocean. Scotland? England?
Somewhere in Europe. Anywhere.

*

In 1991 I travelled to Ireland with Rebecca. I found this big
old house with its warrens of corridors and spooks. Leda came
to live with us, while Keiron, who'd left school and was working in a resort hotel, stayed behind in Arizona. Rebecca
somehow believed I could make it, and she had faith enough to
uproot and take yet another chance on me. It wasn't going to
be easy, she knew that as well as I did. But I'd gone through
the inverted world of drink and drugs and I was infinitely
*weary* of it, and all its torment and devastation and the nuclear
testing-ground I'd made of my mind; in the end self-destruction isn't the big dramatic romantic statement it's trumped
up to be, the last sweet refuge of the creative temperament, a
poetic tomb, flowers heaped against a headstone and a sorry
narcissistic epitaph. Bullshit: it's pathetic. It's also false advertising – destroy yourself, you do more than that; you also
destroy those who have had the strength and courage to love
you, despite your infuriating failings and all the misery you've
shovelled into their lives. Because love endures.

In March 1993 I drank a glass of Guinness in Dublin: my
last to date. I claim no special courage, valour, great will
power, divine intervention. I write this five years later in the
heart of the bog, and the real reason behind my quitting is that
I'm shit-scared of disturbing the demons that hibernate still
inside me; they sleep in the sunken crypts of myself. And
nothing, *nothing*, terrifies me more than riding the passenger
train back to Slipsville, because this time I know it will come
off the rails and go spinning and turning through the air, and
down into some abyss from which there isn't another return.

Two nights ago, before I wrote the above sentences, I
dreamed of Eileen. In this dream Rebecca and I went inside a
restaurant and Eileen was sitting at a table, and she turned to
smile at us. She was about thirty years old and vibrant; she
looked at peace with herself. The image was strong and

somehow very reassuring. *She's young and well again*, I thought. I woke up suddenly, wondering how Eileen might have analysed the dream. I thought vaguely of other dimensions beyond this one; places where our senses are too limited to penetrate.

I saw pale dawn light between the wooden shutters, and I imagined Barbara setting out for Scotland on 31 July 1997, in a mood of fear and hope and a sense of time running out – akin to the feelings in my own heart when I left the United States for Ireland.

Barbara travelled by car to Edinburgh, where she'd made an appointment to visit the General Register Office in Edinburgh. She was accompanied on the five-hour drive from Yorkshire by her friend Netta, a qualified nurse, someone very familiar with Barbara's long search. A day of intermittent sun and rain, and rainbows in the sky ahead of them; all through the Border Country, that soft green lovely landscape England shares with Scotland and yet a land that neither truly owns, the rainbows persisted. Barbara and Netta played old tapes in the car – Elvis, the Beatles – but Barbara's mood was unsettled even as she sang along to familiar tunes. It wasn't just the knowledge of her cancer that troubled her: she was looking forward to the search for Eileen's birth certificate, yet at the same time gearing herself up for more disappointment. Would she come away from Edinburgh empty-handed, as she'd come away from Leeds, as she'd come away so many times before from the offices of Social Services workers? The elusive Eileen – what if this was just another chase after a wild goose? What if there was no trace of the woman? What then? Barbara couldn't imagine where she'd go if Edinburgh proved a wash-out. It was either the dead end of the old trail, or the beginning of a new one. Why anticipate? Why not just listen to the songs and enjoy

the countryside and pretend it was only a day's outing with
an old friend and some comfortingly familiar music? No –
she couldn't make that kind of imaginative leap: she had one
goal, and it wasn't make-believe, and this trip wasn't any
relaxed Sunday afternoon jaunt through the small towns of
the Scottish Borders.

The General Register Office in Edinburgh was located, not
very originally, at New Register House, 3 West Register Street;
the town planner or level-headed councillor who'd named the
house and the street clearly hadn't been given to ornate flights
of fancy. In this government office Barbara and Netta were
directed by a security guard towards what was called the
North Search Room.

This room was equipped with long desks, and each desk
had three or four computers. Barbara, who had no computer
experience, was overwhelmed: what keys did you press? How
did you begin? What if she pressed the wrong keys and systems crashed? She was spooked by electronic instrumentation,
networks, interfacing, all the mysterious terminology and
functions of this whole new world. But sometimes an unexpected kindness comes to one's assistance, even in the cold
heart of a bureaucracy, and Barbara was helped that day by
one of the office assistants, Christine, who had an interest in
searches connected with adoption.

With Christine's aid, Barbara began looking for Eileen's
birth certificate on the computer. She went back through
the years. 1941. 1940. 1939. 1938. She found nothing in '41,
'40, nothing in '39; no record of Eileen's birth in those
years.

Christine tapped the keys for 1938.

And it exploded on the screen suddenly, a copy of the
birth-certificate Barbara had sought for so long: *Eileen Evelyn
Altman, born 5 February 1938, Glasgow.* Finally!

She's real, Barbara thought. She exists. My mother. The girl who carried me for nine months. For the first time in Barbara's life, Eileen Evelyn Altman was more than just a name. Barbara touched the screen with her fingertips, and she cried quietly, aware that people around her were watching her reaction.

The discovery of the birth certificate was a beginning, because now Christine was able to harvest more background information – marriage and death certificates for Doris and Israel, birth certificates for Eileen's brother Sydney, and for Sydney's children too: a family tree had bloomed unexpectedly in the North Search Room of New Register House.

And now the next stage had to be approached, the next task undertaken. What had happened to Eileen? Had she married? Did she have other children?

Or – and this was a harrowing possibility, something to stop Barbara's heart – maybe she'd already died. Maybe she'd been dead for years. This idea was too unbearable to contemplate but Barbara knew she had to keep going, no matter what truth she might find. She was knocking on the door of the secret house in which her mother had always lived – and she couldn't quit now, not until someone opened that door and answered the remaining questions.

So, with grim reluctance, the search for a death certificate began. Barbara started in 1997, and worked slowly backward through forty-two years, to her own birth in 1955, forty-two separate taps of the keyboard, each click another year gone; she felt a deep sense of apprehension as she travelled down through time – maybe she'd come this far only to discover that Eileen had died, which would have been one cruelty too many, a blow to the heart too difficult to take.

Back and back she went, click click click, each click like a nail hammered quietly into a coffin; each click growing louder every time her fingertip made contact with the keyboard. *Please don't be dead*, she thought. *Don't leave me like this. Never having known you, never having a memory of you.*

Back and back. Click and click. Down through the 70s, the 60s. The years rolling away. And then the 50s. *Slow down. Take your time.* 1959, no death certificate. 1958, no death certificate. *A deep breath, Barbara.* 1957, nothing. 1956, nothing. *Only one more year to check.* Barbara hesitated at the year of her birth, 1955. Might Eileen have died in that year? It was possible, in a world that randomly inflicted cancer *anything* was possible, any kind of cruelty and injustice.

She knew she had to tap the key one more time. The screen blurred a little in front of her eyes. One last touch of the keyboard, that was all, and then she'd know. She held her breath and pressed the key.

There was no death certificate for Eileen Evelyn Altman in 1955. *She hadn't died, she was alive, Eileen was alive—*

Barbara was overcome with enormous relief, but it didn't last long, because she realised with a shock that all she'd really established was that her mother hadn't died in *Scotland*. What if she'd emigrated and died in Brisbane or Auckland or Vancouver or Chicago? There would be no record of such a faraway death recorded in Edinburgh. In fact, apart from the birth certificate, there was no other record of Eileen in the Edinburgh computer. No marriage. No children. Not in Scotland anyway.

Barbara's next step was to examine the electoral rolls in Edinburgh's main library. She found no trace of her mother, although she located an address for Eileen's brother Sydney. Sydney would surely know what had become of his sister. He was the key to Eileen.

Barbara and her friend Netta drove back to Yorkshire. *What next?* Netta wanted to know. A tricky question, because although Barbara realised the only answer was to contact Sydney, she wasn't sure how to go about it – cold call him? Write a letter? How were you expected to act in a situation like this? What if Sydney didn't want to speak to her? What if he wouldn't reveal his sister's whereabouts? Imponderables. Barbara, who liked to think things through before she acted, allowed herself a day of quiet contemplation in Yorkshire before she took the next step.

On 2 August 1997, she telephoned Sydney in Glasgow.

When he'd had time to compose himself, Sydney said, 'I'm really very sorry to hear you're ill too. And I don't mean to be difficult, but I think it would be a terrible shock for her if you just phoned her without any warning. She's in hospital in the States, in Phoenix.'

Barbara was derailed by this news of her mother's health. *Eileen had cancer: and she was <u>where</u>? <u>Phoenix</u>? How far away was that? Wasn't that in the desert?* Barbara had never been in the United States. She wasn't sure of the geography of the place. 'Tell me how bad she is.'

'She's had laser surgery, and she's being fed through a tube. Phoning her wouldn't do any good. She couldn't speak even if she wanted to. The cancer's in her lung. Maybe elsewhere too, for all we know.'

Lung cancer. This savage coincidence horrified Barbara: mother and daughter – separated for forty-two years, lives lived apart, different histories, backgrounds – struck by the same disease. She explained to Sydney that her own future was uncertain, and how she'd been looking for Eileen for many years: couldn't he help? Couldn't he do something? Couldn't he please do *something*?

Sydney, genuinely fearful of Eileen succumbing to heart failure if Barbara contacted her directly, told Barbara that the only connection he had with Eileen in her present state was through her friend Nancy Frick, and that he called Nancy every Sunday morning for a health bulletin. He made what he considered a reasonable offer; if Barbara wanted to write a letter, he'd be happy to forward it. He also gave her some brief details about Eileen's life – including the fact that she had three sons, information that delighted Barbara, because all her life she'd considered herself an only child. Suddenly she had three brothers! She wasn't alone. She wondered where they were, and what they looked like, and whether she'd ever see them.

But mainly she wondered if, after all this time, she'd be too late to see her mother.

She wrote a letter:

*Dear Eileen,*

*Thankyou. Thankyou is the one word I have wanted to say to you for over thirty years. People have often asked me how I would feel and what I would say if I ever found you. The answer has been the same for as long as I can remember, that I would feel overwhelming joy in my heart and would want to say 'thankyou' for giving me the gift of life. The news of finding you did give me the joy I had expected, but it was tinged with sadness to find out you are so faraway. I am so desperately sorry to hear about your illness after speaking with Sydney yesterday for the first time.*

*In October last year, I was told my ovaries were in the first stages of cancer. In May this year I was informed that the cancer had spread to my lymph glands and lungs. I am at present receiving a different chemo-drug in the hope that the illness can be put into remission. I sincerely hope that this letter does not impede your recovery, or distress or hurt you in any way.*

*I feel as if my quest has been fulfilled. I have found where you are. However, I am a realistic person and am not under the illusion of a fairy-tale ending. I will respect your decision if you do not want to contact me, although my deepest hope is that you will.*

*I can only end by saying that I hope this letter has gladdened, not saddened you.*

*With all the love I have, I send to you now,*
*Your daughter, Barbara*

She posted this letter to Sydney so that he'd forward it to Phoenix. She waited for two weeks. She heard nothing. She was sinking into a state of numb depression. Two weeks was surely enough time for her mother to have received the letter and answered it . . . if she wanted to. Barbara's first conclusion was that Eileen had no desire to get in touch. She wanted the past to be left alone: *baby? What baby? Oh, I'd almost forgotten all about that time.* Barbara's next thought – her mind was hunting all across an unfamiliar landscape by this time – was that her mother's illness was worse than she'd been led to believe, and Eileen simply wasn't capable of replying. Sometimes silence is the worst kind of news.

Sydney telephoned her two weeks after her initial contact, gave her a progress report on Eileen, said her health was improving. She'd been undergoing radiotherapy, she'd been removed from the feeding tube, but she was still unable to talk. Barbara waited anxiously to hear if there had been any reaction from Eileen to her letter.

Then Sydney lit the fuse of the bomb. 'By the way, I'm holding on to your letter a wee while longer. When I think the time is right, and Eileen's strong enough, I'll forward it. I give you my word on that.'

*He hasn't sent it! He hasn't posted the damn letter!*

Barbara was devastated, shellshocked, barely able to understand what he was telling her; she couldn't believe the letter was
still in Glasgow. She'd imagined it winging across the Atlantic,
reaching her mother, her mother reading it, maybe wondering
how to respond. And now she learned that her hopes and fears
and her two weeks of waiting had been time ruined. She was
sick, for God's sake, her mother was sick – why couldn't the
letter be sent now? Nobody knew how much life either woman
had left. So why the damned delay? Who gave Sydney the right
to be the guardian of his sister's health? He wasn't God, he
couldn't play these kind of games, couldn't come between
mother and daughter unless that was the express wish of
Eileen. Barbara was angry, but didn't want to vent it directly
against Sydney; if she alienated him, he could cut her off, sev-
ering the only link she had to her mother. He controlled the
faucet of information. He could turn it off at any time.

This went on for weeks. Week after week. Seven weeks
total. Seven long unbearable weeks. And still Sydney didn't
send the letter. He always said more or less the same thing:
when she's up to it, when she's back on her feet, I'll do it . . .
He was at least considerate enough to send Barbara photographs of Eileen – the first time Barbara had ever seen her
mother's likeness; looking on the image of the woman whose
life had haunted her for years gave the reality of her mother
added substance.

Although the photographs were priceless, and wonderful to
have, they weren't flesh. And Barbara had lived too long with
her determination to be satisfied with mere pictures. Nick
wondered how she could put up with Sydney's procrastina-
tion. Why hadn't she reached screaming pitch with him? Why
wasn't she more demanding? After all, she was *this* close to her
mother; *one bloody letter away*.

Eight weeks after she'd first contacted Sydney, Barbara's

composure was gone, her nerves fried. She'd been angry, but what was the point of fuming? It achieved nothing. She devised another approach. If Sydney was going to continue putting the decision off, she'd circumvent him. She called information in Phoenix and obtained Eileen's telephone number and address. She'd simply rewrite her letter, she decided, and send it direct to her mother.

She'd force the issue, but at the same time she didn't want to upset Sydney altogether; after all, he was acting in what he believed were Eileen's best interests. She wrote him a letter telling him, in a polite way, she had an address for Eileen, and if he wouldn't forward her original letter, she'd send it herself.

Sydney, cornered, responded to the ultimatum. He telephoned Barbara the next Sunday. This time he reported that he'd sent her letter off to Eileen. He'd also instructed Nancy Frick to prepare Eileen for what was coming in the mail.

Barbara, in a growing state of agitation, could only wait again. What would her mother say when she received the letter? Would she be pleased? Annoyed? Would the letter be an unwanted intrusion? Was Barbara a memory she preferred to avoid? What were the circumstances behind the adoption? The questions – too many of them – rolled back and forth inside her head with the persistence of a tide. She'd come too far to be rebuffed now by her own mother. Surely Eileen would at least be curious to hear from her, perhaps even see her – if there was still time.

Time was the key.

On the night of 21 September 1997, the telephone rang in Barbara's house. She answered. The woman's voice on the line was husky, hesitant. 'Is this Barbara?'

Barbara's answer was a question. 'Is this Eileen?'

Eileen said, 'This is your mother.'

# Part Three

# 17

WHEN Sydney telephoned Nancy Frick to tell her that Barbara had written to Eileen – and that Eileen should be forewarned – he felt he was finally betraying the old family secret. He didn't introduce the subject of Barbara immediately; in fact, he was so nervous and hesitant, his conversation so circuitous, that Nancy had to ask him if he had something on his mind other than his sister's health.

Sydney, making small talk and stumbling over hurdles of words, eventually told the story of the baby and the adoption. It hadn't occurred to him that Eileen, in the normal course of a long friendship with Nancy, would have confided in her the story of the adoption at some point. When Nancy, a little amused by Sydney's discomfort, informed him that she already knew about the adoption saga, that it was ancient history and he didn't have to suffer any embarrassment, he was relieved. He didn't need to go through the whole halting spiel; he was still wary of revealing secrets.

Sydney asked Nancy how, in her opinion, Eileen would take

it when she learned that her daughter wanted to make contact. Nancy's reply was positive and immediate – Eileen would be thrilled, deliriously so: only a few weeks before, she and Eileen had been watching a TV show about reunions of long-lost family members and Eileen had speculated aloud about Barbara, wondering how it would feel if by some miracle she could see her again. I like to think of Eileen remembering, as she looked at TV pictures of relatives being reunited after lifetimes of sad separation, the baby she'd mentally photographed in Scarborough; did she wonder what Barbara looked like now? Did she ever have flights of fancy where she tried to imagine how the baby's face would have changed from infancy to childhood to adolescence to adulthood? Or was Barbara forever a baby in her imagination?

Nancy told Sydney that she'd be more than happy to relay the news of Barbara to Eileen. Sydney, a worrier, was still concerned: was Nancy *sure* about the timing of this? Yes, Nancy was *very* sure about it. Nancy couldn't have been more sure of anything. And even if she'd had *any* residual uncertainty, it was dispelled entirely when Sydney explained that Barbara was also suffering from cancer.

After the phone call, Nancy thought that the news of Barbara reappearing was going to change everything; it would alter the course of Eileen's life. She couldn't wait to break the story – even if she didn't relish the prospect of having to reveal the dark side of it, Barbara's illness. She drove at once to the apartment Eileen shared with Stephen.

Eileen's old lover and friend, Michael, was visiting from Ohio; by yet another of those tiny correspondences that run like a network of veins throughout this story, he was en route for California to seek out his long-lost teenage son. Nancy announced that she wanted to speak in private with Eileen. She made tea and took it into the bedroom and lay down

beside Eileen, and Michael left. Despite her frailty and the
recent surgery and the fact that her voice hadn't fully returned,
Eileen hadn't lost any of her astuteness; cancer hadn't blunted
her instinct. She knew something was going on, and Nancy
hadn't just dropped in to have a cup of tea and a quiet chat.

Nancy took her hand and said that she'd been talking on the
phone with Sydney, who wanted her to relay some news.
Eileen's first thought was that something was wrong in
Glasgow, a family illness, an accident, a dreadful event: there
was an unusual gravity in Nancy's voice.

Nancy said, 'It's about Barbara.'

'Barbara?' Eileen was puzzled a second.

'Your daughter.'

Eileen promptly raised a hand to her heart, and then to her
mouth, and threw back her head and said, '*Oh my God, thank
you thank you,*' and tears streamed across her cheeks and she
couldn't stop crying as she kept saying '*thank you, God, thank
you*' – because apparently she'd prayed for this only a few days
ago, she'd prayed for news of her daughter, and her prayer had
been answered, just like that, just when you least expected an
answer, out there in the vast silence of the universe Somebody
had actually been *listening,* paying attention to the sound of
one lonely voice calling; who would have believed such a thing
possible?

Instantly, the bedroom was abuzz with energy, Nancy
couldn't stop talking about the information she'd gleaned from
Sydney about Barbara, how she was married and had three
kids, Eileen couldn't overcome her astonishment that she'd
not only learned about her daughter's life, but also that she
had three grandchildren she'd known nothing about, it was all
laughter and tears of disbelief and bright Christmas-morning
excitement in that bedroom, and questions – where does
Barbara live? what's her husband's name? how old are the

kids? . . . but Nancy had one more item of news to add, and she was reluctant, because she didn't want to puncture the bubble of Eileen's excitement. But she had no choice. She told Eileen that Barbara was ill. She had cancer, and the cancer had gone into her lungs.

Unexpectedly, Eileen waved the information aside and shook her head dismissively. She wasn't going to be dismayed by this knowledge; no damn way. She was too excited. It was as if the emergence of Barbara from the past had provided her with a booster shot of great energy, or had erected some kind of force-field around her that illness couldn't penetrate. She didn't believe it was any coincidence that Barbara had come into her life at this time; it had to mean something, nothing happened without a reason, at least to Eileen's way of thinking. 'She wants to see me, Nancy. That's the important thing. She wants to see me! *She wants to know me!* And I want to see my daughter. It doesn't matter what shape she's in, or what shape I'm in. We've got to meet. You know what this is, Nancy? It's a gift. It's a great gift.'

The next step, unwrapping the gift, was for Eileen to phone Barbara. Nancy didn't have the number. She had to call Sydney to get it. She gave it to Eileen, who then became hesitant. She picked up the phone, put it down, picked it up again, did this a few times. She was composing in her head what to say, how to begin. So many years were lost and irrecoverable, casualties of separation. Nancy wondered if it might be too late in England to phone anyhow, it was almost midnight there, wait until morning, but Eileen was beyond consideration of time and behavioural protocol – there were no restrictions between mother and daughter, not after such a long absence. No boundaries. Nothing was off-limits now. It was suddenly a world where joy could bloom at the heart of sickness.

She finally dialled the number in Yorkshire, and Barbara answered.

In her journal, Barbara wrote about that first phone call: *Something deep inside of me has been awakened. It's a love I haven't known before. This is the most powerful feeling I have ever experienced. The words 'This is your mother' – these were more intense than the births of my children. One of the first things my mother said was that she hadn't realised how deeply she'd buried the pain and locked it away for forty-two years. And she hadn't looked for me because she feared I'd reject her because I'd blame her for giving me up. I told her I'd never blamed her once. And then we both wanted to know so much about each other, we were interrupting all the time, and crying.*

They conversed at speed, half-finished phrases, overlapping sentences, there was too much to be said, lifetimes to be narrated. They looked for resemblances, small similarities, mother and daughter searching for reflections of themselves in each other. It was as if they needed to find in each other a sense of mutual recognition, a kind of lifebelt they could both grab and share as they were tossed this way and that by the tidal force of the moment. They'd both worked in the health field. Eileen had treated brain-injured kids, Barbara handicapped adults. They talked about their illness, the similarity of symptoms, treatment, side effects. But it was all too draining, too exhilarating. Too many tears. Too many hyper-charged jolts to the heart. Too many things that couldn't be talked about properly during a phone call, and emotions that could only be explored face to face.

During this animated laughing-crying conversation, Barbara's husband and children had been eavesdropping. When finally she hung up forty-five minutes later, Nick hugged her and told her he hadn't ever seen her look this happy before.

Barbara, for her part, was stunned to realise that she'd been speaking to a woman on the other side of the world, one whose face she'd never seen and whose voice she'd never heard, and that this woman, this *stranger*, was her long-lost mother. *She'd missed forty-two of my birthdays,* she wrote, *but for me they all came at once with this one phone call.*

It was wonderful, and it filled Barbara with awe. But it wasn't enough. The telephone was never satisfying. She would have to go to Phoenix and meet Eileen.

# 18

My first reaction to the news that Eileen had spoken with her daughter on the phone wasn't just surprise – oh, God, I don't *believe* it; it was more a sense of astonishment at the weirdness of things, a feeling that maybe, just maybe, some kind of strange order lay under the seemingly whimsical surface of reality. It was as if a bizarre clock ticked at the heart of the universe, one whose mechanism worked in synchronicity very rarely, perhaps only once in anyone's lifetime, and that split second had happened in the lives of Eileen and Barbara, that fragment of time when the hands of the clock come together. Mother and daughter had been lost to each other, and now they were found.

I marvelled at the *ifs* of events – if Barbara hadn't discovered she had cancer, she might not have hurried to Edinburgh when she did. If she'd delayed that trip, the outcome of her life would have been different. If Sydney had been another kind of person, one who wanted total control of access to his sister, he might have told Barbara from the very outset that he'd lost touch with Eileen. Or if he'd been mean-spirited, he could easily have said *sorry, I'm afraid she died some years ago*, and never mentioned Barbara's name to Eileen. If Barbara hadn't been compelled in the first place by the basic demands of the heart to locate her mother, then the hands of the clock wouldn't have stirred at all . . . a chain of ifs.

The boys had different reactions to the news of Barbara's existence. Stephen was overjoyed to discover he had an older sister. He reacted with such fierce happiness that he might have been looking for a Big Sister all his life. Keiron told me later, with a mock-coy smile, that although he was pleased to learn about Barbara, the only thing that 'bothered' him slightly was the fact that his mother hadn't been a virgin when I married her – a small joke, although I wondered if there might be a tiny element of shock or disappointment behind it. I wasn't sure: had Keiron imagined that when his mother met me we were both, so to speak, pure? Keiron, closet romantic, believer in the chaste: this notion struck me as amusing, because when it came to the subject of sex he was candid and outspoken, and often told elaborate and sometimes funny tales of his adventures in Seattle. Iain was deeply involved in exams and so focused on schoolwork that the whole Barbara business was something of a distraction. Later, he'd change this attitude, but at that time he didn't need anything that upset the order of his life. His mother's cancer had already done that. He wanted peace, an existence of almost monastic simplicity, an absence of relationships that were too complex. Stephen and Keiron were in many ways similar to each other, but Iain was unlike either of them.

To Eileen, who spent a lot of time in her wheelchair and longed for a return to her old vitality, Barbara brought not just reconciliation but a renewal of childlike wonder at the happenings of the world; and when you start wondering, where do you stop? She wondered if between them they could smash this cancer they shared. Blitz it. Howitzer it. They could draw strength from each other and forge one big army out of two smaller ones and wage full-scale bloody war against the disease. She and Barbara talked daily on the phone, some-times more than once, encouraging each other, lifting each other, arming themselves for the conflict, while Barbara con-tinued to make plans for the trip to Phoenix.

Eileen was optimistic enough about the fight when she wrote on 6 October to Don Vanouse, a professor of English, an old friend in Oswego, New York: *I have been on an amazing journey, and still travelling. I cannot tell you how exciting it is. My daughter has been searching for me for thirty years. She is overjoyed, and so am I. We talk on the phone every day and it as though we have known each other all along, only the details were missing . . . I am getting stronger every day. Did you know that my daughter also has cancer? I see this whole experience as the door that opens to true healing for both of us.*

*True healing. An open door.* She used a similar phrase in a note to me written around the same time. *Campbell, I feel no more need for the disease. Barbara's entrance into my life has opened a door to a new chapter . . .* She was busy analysing her dreams, which she'd been doing for the past few years as a matter of course. (Before her illness, she'd lectured on dream therapy in Boulder, Los Angeles, Virginia Beach, Boston and London. She'd developed a talent for public speaking, and loved the heady rush she got from talking to groups about the interpretation of dreams. She said it gave her the chance to be the actress she always wanted to be.) She told me she'd dreamed recently of a little garden, prepared for her by her mother. '*I saw there was even a garden hose so I could water the flowers which she had planted for me. The garden represented new growth, and I had the tools to make it grow. The flowers symbolised new and positive thoughts.'* She believed without any doubt that dreams contain meaningful signals, and if she developed these 'new and positive thoughts' she'd be on the high road back to health.

She also accepted without question that her cancer had its origin – not in the pollutants of the everyday world, not in bad diets and insecticides and radioactive fallout from leaky reactors and tobacco, not even in her genetic makeup – but in the pain she'd buried forty-two years before and hauled around with her ever since without pausing to analyse it; it may have been wrapped around with the cobwebs of time, but it was still there under all the intricately structured strands. Now, with Barbara coming to be at her side, she could somehow get well, she'd rid her body of the thing that was eating its way through her. She'd be the living proof of the proposition: we are what we think. Better still: we are what we *refuse* to think.

She was scribbling avidly in notebooks. In one she'd written: *I have much to do and do not feel I have completed what I am here to do. My work at the Clinic isn't quite over yet. I get tremendous joy and satisfaction from my involvement in the lives of the patients who come to the programme. I want to live.*

After her sixth and final Taxol treatment, Barbara's tumour marker test was down, although it seemed to her that her physicians weren't as encouraged by this as she was. They arranged for her to have another scan on 4 October, the week before she was due to fly to the United States, but cancer was the last thing on her mind. She could think of nothing else but the trip, the momentous meeting with Eileen; the prospect overwhelmed her, consumed her. Having spent so much time digging in the past, now she was living in the immediate future. She was going forward, not back.

Along with the daily phone calls between the two women, photographs were exchanged; Eileen got to see the grandchildren she'd never met, and Barbara the younger brothers she was still to encounter. Barbara's three children had also spoken to their 'new' grandmother on the telephone; the flow of information traffic – letters, e-mails, calls – was heavy. As the time for departure drew closer, Barbara couldn't eat, sleep, she was fuelled mainly by the adrenaline of anticipation.

Financially the trip was a burden, because Nick had no income other than disability benefits from an old work-related accident, and Barbara wasn't fit to continue nursing; there weren't enough funds for husband and two sons to travel, although they were able to scrape sufficient money together for Heidi to accompany her mother – who was certainly in no condition to travel alone. Barbara's friend Netta also wanted to make the trip; she'd been following Barbara's search for a long time, and naturally didn't want to be excluded from the denouement. Another friend, Judith – Jude – whom Barbara had known for thirty years, wanted to come along too. Judith, a fair-haired slim woman of about fifty, was a community services worker who specialised in home-care aid. Like Netta, she'd been intrigued by Barbara's prolonged quest. They'd both lived through Barbara's various disappointments in the past – the cold trails, the leads that faded out, the harsh disappointments, the obduracy of bureaucrats. Both women shared something else too, a concern for Barbara's health, the worry that she might be driving herself too hard; and they wondered what they'd do if her health took a serious downward turn in Arizona – a long way from the physicians who knew her case.

On the night of 10 October, Barbara called Eileen four or five times – she couldn't rest, couldn't relax, she was in ecstatic disarray, couldn't believe she was actually making this trip,

6000 miles to see her mother – *my mother*, how strange and wonderful those two commonplace words seemed – the whole situation wasn't real, it felt like she'd won first prize in a competition she couldn't remember ever having entered, her mind raced and buzzed as if flying in advance of the aeroplane that would eventually take her all the way to Arizona. She was sorry to be leaving Nick and her sons behind, but there wasn't an alternative. And besides, they knew her, they understood. She didn't need to make apologies.

Early on the morning of 11 October, all four women undertook the journey from Yorkshire to London, a four-hour drive; at Heathrow they boarded a United Airlines flight for Chicago, where there would be a five-hour stopover before the connection to Phoenix. Barbara felt no fatigue, unlike her travelling companions, all of whom dozed in the lounge at O'Hare Airport. She'd reached that state of excitement which seems to have no end to it, it's fixed, there's no anti-climax on the other side of it. How could she sleep? She flicked through magazines without seeing them. She walked up and down impatiently. She studied the Arrivals and Departures boards. She browsed through airport shops. Killing time. Waiting. Thinking of the moment when she'd come face to face with Eileen. Four hours' flying time from Chicago to Phoenix.

Now and then Heidi would open her eyes and ask *Are you OK?* or *Is everything all right?* And Barbara would nod and say yes, everything was fine, better than fine. Eventually the boarding call was announced for the flight to Phoenix; the women took their seats. Barbara was light-headed but not jet-lagged. She might have closed her eyes from time to time, but she didn't sleep. Time dragged. Four hours, how could four bloody hours seem so damnably *long*?

Sixty minutes from Phoenix she went inside one of the toilets, washed, changed her clothes. She stared at herself in the mirror and worried about what she saw. She wished she looked more like her old self to meet her mother – strong and healthy, with the thick black curly hair she used to have. And she was forty pounds heavier since she'd started chemotherapy, steroids and the hormone replacement therapy. She was wearing a headscarf because her hair had all but gone, even her eyebrows and lashes had disappeared. She scrutinised her face in the mirror and saw how puffy her eyes were and how dark the circles under them. She pinched her cheeks in a feeble attempt to give herself some colour. She wondered what Eileen would think of her.

Her friend Netta thought that Barbara looked 'rather lovely'. With that Yorkshire flair for unadorned language, Netta felt that if people couldn't see beyond the hair loss and the weight gain, it was just 'tough shit'.

Barbara went back to her seat and tried to relax. When the pilot announced that the plane would shortly be landing at Sky Harbor in Phoenix, Barbara could see the yellow and orange lights of the city and how they stretched away into the vast surrounding desert. And then there was touchdown, the iffy moment of wheels thudding tarmac, followed by the awkward shuffling around of weary passengers in the narrow aisles, and the gathering of hand luggage, and the jet-lagged mumbling of Jude and Netta and Heidi, and the insufferable wait for the plane to taxi to the terminal building, slow, always slow; Barbara wanted to disembark at once, to *leap* out – how much longer now? And then they were off the aircraft and moving along narrow corridors towards the arrivals lounge, Heidi a few steps ahead of her mother. It was Heidi who first spotted Stephen waiting; she recognised him from one of the photographs Eileen had sent.

Barbara thought: *this is my first sight of one of my young brothers*, a perception she barely had time to accommodate before Stephen laughed and grabbed and hugged her, welcoming her – not to Phoenix, not to America, but into his family and his life. Barbara experienced a strong sense of familiarity; it was as if she'd seen Stephen before, met him at some other time, even if she knew this couldn't be. The ghost of a family resemblance perhaps – a little echo of herself in Stephen's features, his eyes, his mouth. She wasn't sure. She just knew there was an instant affinity with him. No awkwardness, no nervousness: she thought, *this is my brother and he's telling me he's happy I've come home*.

'Mom's at the apartment,' Stephen said. 'She's waiting for you.'

'Please take me to her,' Barbara said. 'Take me to my mother.' These were words she never imagined she'd get to say.

In her wheelchair, Eileen waited alone in the apartment. She'd discussed with Barbara the idea of going to the airport to meet her, but she felt the excitement would be too much for her and she'd have to resort to using her portable oxygen tank (which she hated, it drew stares from people, looks of curiosity or sometimes sympathy), and in any case she didn't want her first view of Barbara to be from a wheelchair; a half-mast view, was how she described it. So she waited, and she thought of Scarborough, and the wild tides of winter, and how she'd walked along the promenade with her father – dead for such a long time now – and how she'd given away her baby; and she asked herself, What will I feel? What will it be like to hold her again?

She studied the photographs Barbara had sent from Yorkshire. Barbara as an infant, a young girl, a woman. She cried as she gazed at these pictures. *I missed all this*, she thought. *All her growing up. I wasn't there for her. I have carried*

*her inside myself somewhere for forty-two years. I've lived with*
*her embalmed within me. A baby frozen in time.*
*And now she's coming back to me.*

She'd wondered about the first contact: should she stay in
the bedroom and wait until she and Barbara were alone before
they talked? Or would it be better to go outside to the patio
and be there when Stephen brought Barbara from the airport?
Before she could decide, she heard a car draw up, and she got
out of her wheelchair and walked to the glass door that led
from the living room to the patio. Her heart was topsy-turvy
and her legs shook, but she was as prepared as she'd ever be.

Stephen parked his six-seater van, which was crammed with
people and luggage, and rushed inside to announce Barbara's
arrival – 'She's here, she's here, are you ready for this, Mom?' –
and then hurried back out to the vehicle again, telling Barbara
to come indoors. She got out of the van and walked through a
gate in a cedar fence into the small patio area at the rear of the
apartment.

And there, standing just outside the door, was her mother.
She was thin, pale, dressed in a blue T-shirt and loose-fitting
white pants, her red hair cut short and brushed neatly. She
stood under a pale lamp. An overwhelming moment: without
hesitation, without awkwardness, without words, the two
women clutched each other in a flurry of tears and happiness,
and relief. Barbara experienced a deep feeling of love; the
bond that occurred between Eileen and herself was instant,
high voltage. Immediately, she felt secure, loved. Whole. She'd
found her blood-ties. She'd found the place where she
belonged: her mother's arms. All her life had been leading to
this moment of reconciliation.

Everyone else around faded into the background, where
they existed only as indeterminate shadows – Heidi, Barbara's

two friends, Stephen. Eileen and Barbara, mother and daughter, might have been the only two people in the world for that moment. Weeping, Eileen pulled back from the embrace briefly. There was a tremble in her hoarse voice, a catch at the back of her throat. 'Let me look at you. Is this *really* my baby?'

'Yes,' Barbara said. 'Is this *really* my mum?'

And they held each other again tightly.

After a moment, Eileen broke away and went indoors and picked up from the coffee table a vase containing a red rose. She gave it to Heidi, her granddaughter, as a token of love. Heidi was going through various emotions – she was overjoyed to see her mother and grandmother embrace with such feeling, she felt privileged to be present at so moving a time, she was content that the end of a long quest had been completed.

Then Eileen conjured up a second vase, which contained two red roses. She gave this to Barbara.

'A symbol of reunion,' Eileen said.

Still crying, Barbara took the flowers and thought how long and how hard it had been to find Eileen and forge this reunion; and now she had no intention of ever letting her mother go.

I have a photograph on my office wall of that first encounter between Eileen and Barbara, that first glad embrace. Barbara has her back to the camera, her face is unseen; she's wearing a black blouse with a white flower pattern and a matching headscarf. Eileen's face is visible, though; her eyes are half-shut and slightly swollen and red from tears, and her expression is one that might be relief, or a gratitude too great to utter, and her thin hands are spread across Barbara's back as she clasps her daughter tightly, as if she means to hold on to her forever, and never lose her again.

# 19

On that first night Nancy Frick, impatient to meet Barbara, visited for a time and then drove the jet-lagged Netta and Judith to her house a few miles away, where accommodation had been arranged for them. Heidi collapsed almost at once on a camp bed set up in a corner of Eileen's bedroom.

An hour after her arrival, Barbara found herself alone with Stephen and Eileen, eating Chinese food Stephen had picked up from a nearby restaurant. Stephen kept laughing in his infectious way, shaking his head and saying, 'This is amazing, this is an *amazing* time.' He hadn't yet absorbed the fact of having a long-lost sister. Eileen, her expression incredulous, held Barbara's hand constantly.

Barbara felt the same sense of disbelief as her mother and brother. Twenty-four hours ago she'd been in her house in Yorkshire, surrounded by the familiar – the street of small well-kept houses where she lived, the neighbours, the local shops, her husband. Now all that was thousands of miles away. She'd been anticipating this experience for weeks, but nothing in her imagination had prepared her for the reality of *being* in

Arizona. So much to take in, so many new impressions and people she hadn't seen except in photographs. She was unable to keep her eyes from her mother's face, except to glance now and again at Stephen: the situation had the timbre of a sweet dream, a sensation compounded by the fatigue of her long journey and the fact she was running on rapid-burning raw adrenaline. Everything was a little unreal, but strangely wonderful. Touching Eileen's hand, looking at her, thinking how vibrant she seemed, Barbara was overjoyed.

There were questions she longed to ask, and mysteries she yearned to solve, but these could wait. She had ten days ahead of her. For the moment talk was restricted to the humdrum – she described the flight, her family and home in Yorkshire, while Eileen chatted about her own sons, and Stephen told stories about his three kids. It was ice-breaking conversation, under the surface of which there were depths to be explored. For now it was enough for Barbara and Eileen to be in the same room. Words were irrelevant; language wasn't adequate.

But reality couldn't be kept outside the door forever – it gatecrashed in the chilly form of small oxygen cylinders placed here and there around the living room, and a large oxygen concentrator inside the bedroom, and Eileen's wheelchair, all reminders of illness. Barbara thought of the years she'd spent searching – how long did she have with her mother now? How much life remained to them? Questions best left unasked: enjoy what you have, she thought. Forget the oxygen and the damn wheelchair and the illness.

When it finally came time to discuss where Barbara would sleep, Eileen suggested she share her double bed. The apartment had only one bedroom, and Stephen had the sofa bed in the living room. Barbara felt awkward; it wasn't the prospect of sleeping with a mother who was still a stranger that made her uneasy – on the contrary, sharing a bed with Eileen struck her as completely natural. It was her own appearance, the fact she'd have to remove her headscarf and reveal her lack of hair, and show the soft babylike down that covered her scalp – this embarrassed her. It was a small hurdle of vanity she had to get over sooner or later.

'You better prepare yourself,' she said, and slowly took off the scarf. 'You won't believe it looking at me now, but my hair used to be dark and thick. The chemo made it all fall out. I got a wig, but I never wear it, I hate it. I prefer this fluff . . .'

Eileen was quick to sense her daughter's discomfort. She stroked Barbara's head and said, 'I remember this head, you know. The last time I saw you, your hair was just like this . . .'

*The last time I saw you.* Barbara was moved by the words and the accompanying gesture. She wrote in her journal: *She often strokes my head. It's the most comforting feeling, a childlike sense of security. I relish these moments. They're precious, very precious.*

Ten days: it wasn't such a long time when you compared it with forty-two years. Ten days of her mother wasn't going to be enough, a scratching of the surface at best. Ten *years* might not be enough. But Barbara would use every moment of her time in Phoenix to get to know Eileen. There were ordinary things to do, mother-daughter things that had been denied them by circumstance – shopping together, cooking together, experiences so normal and everyday that nobody gives them a thought. Simple stuff, scrambling eggs at the stove together, going down the aisles of a supermarket, the banalities of life that in some circumstances turn out to be unexpectedly resonant.

This was a remarkable time for Eileen too. She'd emerged from her recent melancholy slump and she was feeling better, eating well, she had a light in her eye, more energy than before; she'd come a long way from the gaunt frightened worn-out woman in the nursing home in late July. Barbara's emergence had transformed her, even if she still had to use the wheelchair to get around, and was obliged to carry a portable cylinder of oxygen, because she was prone to breathlessness and fits of coughing.

But she had enough enthusiasm to devise lists of goals that consisted of such activities as 'daily breathing exercises', 'get massage once a week'. I have several of her lists on my desk as I write this on a sunny-cold Irish morning.

Under the heading Fun Things, she wrote 'one movie a week', 'cook a new dish', 'sit in the sun for an hour a day'. They were tiny goals. Small objectives. The sick are denied complex endeavours; life becomes a series of simple events, like making a column of wooden building blocks. Triumphs lie in little things. *Cook a new dish*. I imagine her leafing the pages of a culinary magazine or recipe book and wondering what to make – Wild mushroom pie? Asparagus risotto? Shrimp in filo pastry? No, these would be too elaborate for Eileen, whose cooking was never fancy – and whether she had energy enough to get ingredients from the market. But Barbara was here now. Barbara would help. Together, they might complete some of these projects.

Another list I have consists of the stuff Eileen ingested on a daily basis. These were allegedly beneficial substances:

| | |
|---|---|
| Deprenyl | 2mg |
| Recancostat | Follow protocol |
| Flaxseed Oil | 1 tablespoon daily |
| Lecithin | 1 teaspoon |
| Essiac Tea | 1 cup |
| Castor Oil Pack | Nightly |
| Charred Oak Keg | Daily as needed |

Recancostat? Charred Oak Keg? Essiac Tea? Laser therapy

and radiation treatment had left her drained, so why *should* she put her trust in conventional medicine? It had kept her alive, sure, but it hadn't cured her, and what quality of life would it allow her? So why not try strange potions and visualisations and will power? Why not inhale the fumes of magic powders thrown on open flames? Why not believe in unlikely panaceas? You're in the foxhole of cancer, what do you turn to for comfort and sustenance? And why shouldn't Barbara, whose appearance was magical in itself, be a part of the cure?

They went out together, mother and daughter, in the warm October sunshine of Phoenix. Barbara wheeled Eileen through stores or sat with her beside the pool in the apartment complex. Sometimes, for the hell of it, Stephen would whiz Eileen in her wheelchair at speed down supermarket aisles, which she loved, dramatically feigning a sense of panic.

Barbara developed a special relationship with Stephen, whom she had to hit with cushions before he'd respond reluctantly to the alarm clock in the morning; pillow fights with her brother, Stephen getting into the spirit of it and complaining to Eileen, 'Mom, she's hitting me,' and Barbara saying, 'He started it,' and Eileen scolding them with, 'Children, children, behave yourselves.' There was laughter in the mornings in a home that needed fun. It was everyday family life; it just happened to have been delayed by more than four decades.

Eileen slipped into the mood of it all with ease and gratitude and humour. One morning, when she was scolding Barbara for some feigned misbehaviour, she said, 'God, Barbara, I left you alone for two minutes and you didn't come home for forty-two years.'

Barbara decided she wanted to give her mother a new look, so she bought styling combs, and they sat on the edge of Eileen's bed while Barbara brushed her mother's hair. (I imagine the distinctive sound of bristle through hair, that lazy sweeping feminine noise, the intimacy of it.) Eileen gazed at herself in the mirror while Barbara worked with brush and combs, and she said, 'This is what I've missed, Barbara, this girlie stuff, makeup and hair-talk. You need a daughter for these things. Sons are wonderful, but they don't meet all your needs. They don't have . . .' and she searched for the word she wanted . . . 'the *tenderness* of women.'

I like to think Eileen remembered her dream of 'helping hands' coming out of the sky; I like to believe that she looked at Barbara standing behind her in the mirror and realised the hands in her dream belonged to her daughter.

It was an uplifting time, and the repercussions of cancer for a while were shelved and ignored. There was normality of a sort. Barbara felt increasingly drawn to her mother: there had never been anything but ease from the very beginning, but now she realised there was sufficient rapport between them for her to approach the subjects she'd worried over for most of her life.

One night, when they were lying in bed (Heidi had decamped to Nancy's after the first night, because the sound of the oxygen concentrator kept her awake), Barbara raised the matter of her father, although she was hesitant. She didn't want to dig up frightening or horrific memories for her mother.

'Can you tell me anything about him? Only if it isn't too difficult for you . . .'

'It's not difficult at all,' Eileen said. 'He was called Bill, he was eleven years older than me. I was only sixteen when I first met him and completely impressionable. He reminded me of the young Orson Welles, the one from *The Third Man* and *The Lady from Shanghai* – he was brooding and soulful and romantic. I fell madly in love with him. My parents knew nothing about this affair. They would have killed me if they'd found out.'

Barbara was totally baffled. *Bill? Orson Welles?* What was all this stuff about a secret love affair? Seeing her daughter's perplexed look, Eileen asked if there was something wrong.

Barbara answered, 'The story I always heard was that you'd been raped, and that was why you gave me away.'

'*Raped?*' Eileen kissed Barbara's forehead and squeezed her hand reassuringly. 'I wasn't *raped*, dear. You weren't the product of violence. Is that what you've always believed?' In tears suddenly, Eileen held her daughter's head against her breast, gently stroking her face with one hand. 'You were the product of love, Barbara.' And she rocked Barbara quietly in her arms for a moment.

Barbara was astonished, swamped with relief; a burden had been lifted. All those years she'd considered herself a rape baby – and now here was Eileen telling her that her father was a man she'd *loved*. The assault had never happened.

'So where did the rape story come from?' Barbara asked.

Eileen had no trouble answering that. 'It was probably something my mother dreamed up to tell the adoption agency. It made my pregnancy seem more . . . respectable. Something that wasn't *my* fault. She meant well.'

Barbara asked, 'What happened to Bill?'

'He said the baby wasn't his. He was the jealous type anyway. I never saw him again after I told him I was pregnant.'

Barbara wanted to know more. 'What about the time you spent in Scarborough? What was that like?'

Eileen recreated the story of Doris and Issy's fictional world, the walks along the beach, the bacon sandwiches she'd been allowed to eat. She talked fondly about the big room with the piano. 'You and I spent a lot of time together at that piano. That was my special time with you.'

Barbara felt a rush of emotion at her mother's memory; she pictured an image of a young girl all alone picking out tunes on a piano in a large empty room; she thought of how a baby is linked to her mother even *before* birth. How she had been linked to Eileen.

And then Eileen said, 'There's something I want to show you.'

She tugged down the waistband of her trousers to show the scar of her C-section. 'That's been my reminder of you, Barbara. That's the scar you left. You were a Caesarean delivery.'

It was a moment of enormous poignancy for both women. Awed, Barbara looked at the faded wrinkled line, and ran her finger gently across it, delicately; touching the scar reinforced her sense of physical attachment to her mother. It was the definitive seal, the ultimate connection: Eileen had been cut open by a surgeon's knife for Barbara to be born.

Keiron flew in from Seattle to meet his new sister. He hadn't been in Phoenix since July, when he'd stayed with me at the Embassy suites. Eileen was looking forward to his arrival; she wanted him to see how she'd improved since the last time. More, she wanted him to meet Barbara. The encounter was good, brother and sister hugging. Like Stephen, Keiron enjoyed the idea of discovering he had an older sister, and long after Barbara had returned to England he kept in touch with her by telephone, sharing stories of his life in Seattle with her – which always involved the complexities of juggling various girl-friends, and the vicissitudes of forming a rock band.

Barbara, excited at the idea of meeting her youngest brother, nevertheless experienced a sort of sadness: Keiron was seventeen years her junior, the same age difference between herself and Eileen. She was old enough to be his mother. She thought of time elapsed, time forever lost, all the years that were like precious items pawned and no longer redeemable. What had her brothers been like as little kids? She'd missed out on them growing up, their transition from childhood to adolescence, the hundreds of small shared things that constitute relationships, the buzzwords, the family secrets, the in-jokes, the whole emporium of common memories. She'd lost out on Christmases and birthdays and holidays, as well as tonsillectomies and chickenpox and measles. But she belonged, no matter what she'd missed. She was the sister who'd been away for a while, that was all. And the only family member who hadn't shown up yet to welcome her was Iain, a fact that disappointed Eileen.

Iain was Iain, though, and Eileen understood him, and because she knew him she forgave him. As conservative and quiet as Stephen was gregarious, as private as Keiron was public, he needed time to process his thoughts and feelings. He'd come to meet Barbara when he was ready.

He explained his initial adverse response to Barbara's sudden appearance in a note he wrote me: *I'm resentful because Mom could have mentioned Barbara before. We are a very easy-going family and I would have understood. I'm juggling school and helping Mom and the heat is hellish and how I dread the sound of my pager going off and I really don't want to meet any additional family members who just appear out of nowhere.*

I sometimes wondered if he'd been affected by the wound of my divorce from Eileen more than the other two boys, if it had poisoned him in some way; didn't the firstborn have a special place, first claim on the attentions of his parents? Didn't he feel it more when his parents broke up? I also wondered if he nurtured a resentment against the new life I'd created in Ireland with a woman who wasn't his mother, if he felt that his loyalty to Eileen would somehow be compromised if he befriended Rebecca. Keiron accepted Rebecca, and so eventually had Stephen: but Iain was the hold-out, the last to express affection, and even then it didn't come easy to him.

Abrasive emotions sometimes surfaced more quickly for him than gentler ones. Once, in an ice-cream parlour in Scottsdale, he saw Charles Keating, the architect of the great Lincoln Thrift scam that had plundered the life savings of thousands of ordinary people. I was astonished by the way Iain was moved to volcanic rage when he recognised Keating. 'That bastard should be in *jail*,' he spluttered. 'Look at him – what the hell is wrong with this country when guys like that can walk around at liberty? You got any idea what he *stole* from people? And look at the sonofabitch sitting there eating goddamn ice cream!'

I thought for a moment I'd have to restrain Iain, probably the least physically combative person I know, from confronting Charlie Keating and perhaps smashing the bowl of ice cream directly into the fraud's face. But he calmed down eventually. I was impressed by the way an injustice had enraged him, and by the insight I'd been given, quite unexpectedly, into how deeply he felt about certain things. I wondered if he felt at this same level of intensity about a whole range of matters, some of them too complex to express, and others too difficult to admit.

With Nancy Frick's help, a party was arranged to introduce Barbara to Eileen's friends and colleagues at the clinic – physicians, therapists, counsellors; the affair was to be held at the social centre in the community where Nancy lived. Nancy, and to a lesser extent Eileen, had been working the phone energetically for days, setting up this celebration. Excitement, coloured balloons, tables spread with food prepared by Nancy and Judith and Netta, Keiron and Stephen in attendance (Iain absent), the buzz of a special event.

Eileen arrived at the centre dressed entirely in white, looking informal and relaxed. She floated from one group of guests to another, happy, laughing, telling everyone the remarkable story of how Barbara, also stricken with cancer, had appeared in her life; this was what Eileen enjoyed, this was her element, the buzz of storytelling, the dramatic pauses, punchlines, her face expressive, her body animated, occupying the spotlight where she might forget her illness. Guests were touched and moved by the tale of mother and daughter – there were tears and laughter and photographs, and Barbara was introduced to more people than she could ever hope to remember. She watched her mother flit here and there without the assistance of either a wheelchair or oxygen; Eileen drew her energy from the event, the delight of her friends, the sense of occasion. And with each telling of her story she looked at Barbara with fierce, almost possessive pride, as if she wanted to say *Thank you, kid, for turning up when you did. You've given me far more than just a damn good tale to tell people. You've given me the kind of therapy no doctor can give.*

There is a photograph of Eileen taken when she was about ten years of age; its colours are paled a little by time, but you can still tell that her hair is red. She's dressed for ballet class. The picture is posed – she's in a dancer's stance, and she's smiling directly into the camera. What's obvious from this long-ago shot is that she loved the camera, she adored the idea of a lens being focused on her and having her image trapped, somewhat theatrically, on celluloid. Many of her photographs are similar; she's mugging for the camera, showing off, inhibitions shoved aside, she's just having fun.

On the day of the party, this was the Eileen that re-emerged, the one who liked to have her photograph taken, the good sport, the storyteller, the healthy lively woman. She was in coruscating form. How good she must have felt that afternoon, how in touch with life and well-being! As she went from person to person, table to table, she might have shed years as well as her sickness. Cancer? You've got the wrong lady, guys. There's nothing wrong with me. She had Barbara and Heidi in tow, both of whom were being hugged by everyone they met, no handshakes here, no Brit-style reserve, this is a country of huggers . . . it was a freewheeling time, high-spirited, and Eileen made it from one o'clock until five o'clock, without coughing or becoming breathless.

When she got home that evening, she was happy and content. The day had gone brilliantly. Her friends had all shown genuine affection to Barbara, and to Heidi. If only some days could last forever. If only that day had been preserved in amber; if only the world had come to a dead halt on that one particular Saturday in October 1997; decay and disease would have been arrested, all would have been well.

But time moves on, and cancer, that relentless stalker, isn't still; even when you feel good, as Eileen did that evening, it's only because the watcher in the shadows is taking a break, building up strength, working up thirst.

The day following the party, a trip was made to Sedona to view the spectacular Red Rock scenery. An eight-seater van was hired, and along with another van that belonged to Stephen's wife, fifteen people (Eileen, the boys, Stephen's family, Nancy and her two teenage kids, and Barbara and Heidi, Netta and Judith) travelled north in these two vehicles to Red Rock country, about seventy miles north of Phoenix. For Stephen and Keiron, both of whom had lived here for a time with Rebecca and myself, the trip was nostalgic; familiar rocky landmarks, the scenes of outrageous all-night outdoor keggers and bonfires, the place where Keiron almost drove a Volkswagen off a cliff.

Barbara and Keiron, who travelled in the same vehicle, spent time catching up with each other's lives, talking about schooldays, work, likes, dislikes. They compared hands and discovered their fingers were exactly the same length and shape. Why not? Brother and sister, resemblances. Keiron was thrilled to discover that when they made faces, each was able to duplicate precisely the other's distorted appearances. They sang songs (Keiron, like Eileen, wasn't blessed with a great voice; a drawback of sorts for a musician) and behaved like little kids – an escape into childishness, freedom from anxiety, a short release from stressful thoughts of a future that might be unbearable. The sun burned on the red rocks, the sky was the blue of a god's eye, the fall scenery dappled.

At lunchtime the whole gang went to a restaurant. As she picked at her food, Barbara realised how transient the situation was; she had only a few more days left before her return to Yorkshire. She didn't want to leave her mother. The time in Eileen's company had gone too quickly, and she wanted more. How could she simply pack a suitcase and fly away after only ten days? This feeling was amplified by the fact that Keiron was returning that night to Seattle, his brief visit over. Things were coming apart, the relationships she'd developed, the family she'd found, people would go their separate ways and everything become diluted by distance and absences – or so she felt as she looked across the table at her mother, who winked and asked her if she was OK. But she wasn't OK and she didn't look OK, she was on a downward spiral, and Eileen sensed it. And so did Keiron, who made her a spontaneous gift by working a paper napkin into the shape of a flower (he has a knack for this kind of party trick) and passing it to her. The offering cheered her for a while, but the clouds were gathering at the back of her head.

On the return to Phoenix and the airport, where Keiron had to catch his plane, her gloom grew. Eileen knew, and held her hand reassuringly. 'It's OK to be sad, Barbara. It's OK to feel sorry when somebody leaves,' she said.

Barbara barely had time to hug Keiron and exchange addresses and phone numbers before he hurried inside the great insensate maw of the terminal building. She watched him go, and she thought: *snap out of this mood. Step off this treadmill of depression.* She had to be more positive, because any negative feelings would affect Eileen, and the last thing Barbara wanted was to deflate her mother's new-found vivacity, this fresh lease she appeared to have negotiated with that most demanding of landlords – Life.

But time was against Barbara, and before long she'd be back in her own home. It was as if she had two lives now, two homes; a person divided. She'd go back to Yorkshire, there was never really any question about that, she'd go back to her family and that wonderful wild landscape of dales and moors and mists and rain, old coalmines long since closed down and drystone walls enclosing fields, and small villages with their pubs and their ale and their Melton Mowbray pork pies and Cumberland sausages – but an essential part of her would remain behind in Phoenix with her mother.

On the day before she was scheduled to leave, Barbara accompanied Eileen and Nancy to the hospital where Eileen was due to receive the results of a chest scan she'd undergone a week before to check the results of her radiation treatment. Eileen was confident; she'd been feeling fine for days, and you didn't feel this good unless you were on the mend.

In the waiting room at the hospital, Barbara watched her mother reading magazines, thinking how relaxed she seemed. There was no sign of anxiety, no uneasiness. After a short time, Eileen was called by a nurse into a small consulting room. Barbara and Nancy accompanied her. The physician hadn't arrived. Barbara felt tense: she wanted to hear the doctor say, *everything's looking good, radiation's worked wonders, I'm delighted, I wish I had news like this for my patients every day.* But the doctor was taking a long time to appear.

Eileen said, 'I need to pee, and if I wait any longer I won't be able to control myself.' In any other situation, the remark might have gone unnoticed, but here, in the tension of the cramped consulting room awaiting a physician's verdict, it provoked laughter. Nancy and Barbara began to giggle. 'Behave yourselves,' Eileen said. 'We're in a hospital, for heaven's sake.' Her feigned scolding only caused more laughter; none of the three women could restrain themselves. Eileen was laughing harder than the others, so hard in fact that she did pee herself. Levity, lightness of heart, a touch of absurdity – the women needed a few minutes of silliness.

The doctor entered eventually, just as the women regained some form of composure. He asked Eileen to accompany him to another office; he invited Nancy and Barbara to come along, if they wanted. They entered what looked like an upmarket consulting room, big leather chairs, leather-topped executive desk, no examination couch. Pinned to fluorescent screens on the wall were the scan pictures. The physician beckoned the women over to look at them. Barbara stared at the lung area and realised, with a sickening sensation, that it was bad. From her own experience both as nurse and patient, she knew what the doctor was going to tell Eileen. Immediately, she stepped behind Eileen and, slipping her arms around her from the back, she grasped her mother's wrists to give support against the shock that was coming.

The doctor sighed and said, 'I wish I had better news for you.' He told her the cancer was widespread throughout both lungs. Internal radiation wasn't an option. He wanted Eileen to see an oncologist and discuss chemotherapy, but he wasn't optimistic about the usefulness of that treatment.

Eileen buckled as if she'd been struck by a small mine

detonating in her face, and would have collapsed to the floor if Barbara hadn't been holding her. Strength went out of her body completely, suddenly; she was limp and uncoordinated, her spine giving way, all her balance gone. She moaned, then whispered, 'Oh no, God, no.'

There was a short terrifying silence in the room. Basically, Eileen had just heard her own death sentence. Barbara understood what her mother was feeling, but what could she do or say? What kind of consolation or encouragement could she offer Eileen? What could *anyone* say? Language is elastic, but limited; and the deeper the feelings to be described, the more stretched out of shape our language becomes. Barbara thought, *I want to make it all go away for her, but I can't.* She could feel what her mother was going through, and it echoed inside her, that grim terror when the news is unbearably bad, that abyss of total fear, that fall through endless space, through total silence, not even the slightest whimper of a wind in your ears. Down and down and down, dying; a last sunset, a last layer of light fading.

Eileen recovered enough to ask the doctor what happened next, where did she go from here? The physician answered that she should think about receiving care from the Hospice movement, which would provide pain relief as the illness got worse; in all likelihood, the cancer would spread to the bone. It may have done so already.

Eileen was quiet for a while before gathering herself together with what must have been a massive effort of will. Then she said, 'I'm sorry, Doctor. I can't accept your opinion. I feel too *well*.' And she hugged the surprised physician.

It was the end of any further conventional treatment. The only road open to her now was the one she'd already begun to travel, the alternative route, the homeopathic, the holistic; she was still in the foxhole, but it was deeper than before.

\*

Iain finally appeared on the night before Barbara's departure; he hadn't called in advance to say he was coming. He just showed up. He was introduced to Barbara, whom he embraced shyly. He didn't stay long, he chatted inconsequentially, and then kissed his mother and left, saying he'd probably call to say goodbye in the morning. He never did. Eileen explained to Barbara that any embrace from Iain was to be considered something of an 'honour' – he wasn't a toucher; but it was a good sign, and it meant that she was halfway to being accepted by him.

And then it was time to go. Stephen, who had to work and couldn't make the airport run, embraced his sister for a long time on that last morning; neither said goodbye to the other. As he drove away, he blew Barbara a kiss. Barbara found *his* farewell difficult enough, but she dreaded even more the parting from her *mother*. She was coming undone inside, but she'd hide it as best she could for Eileen's sake.

Nancy drove the group to the airport. Judith and Netta said goodbye to Eileen, reaching down to hug her in her wheelchair before they walked towards the flight gate. This left Barbara and Heidi alone in the crowded departure lounge with Eileen and Nancy. Heidi leaned over to receive an embrace from Eileen. And then Eileen looked at Barbara, who was beginning to experience the oncoming panic of departure, the sorrow of finally stepping away and leaving this sick woman she loved.

Eileen said, 'For you, I'll have to stand up,' and she rose slowly to her feet. And just as Barbara, awaiting the last embrace, was about to succumb to tears, Eileen stared around the crowded lounge and cried out, 'I CAN WALK! I CAN WALK! IT'S A MIRACLE! I'M CURED!'

Her voice upraised, she appeared jubilant, triumphant, creating a commotion that caused people to strain through the crowd in the lounge for a sight of this bizarre occurrence. What kind of melodramatic stunt had just been pulled by that thin tiny woman in the wheelchair? Was she crazy or something? Some kinda nut? Maybe out on a day-release programme and due back in her padded room by nine PM, something like that? Eileen understood perfectly well what she was doing, defusing the emotion of the situation, taking the sting out of the farewell, easing her own and Barbara's sorrow; and the fact that it gave her the chance to perform for a captive audience was probably a temptation too overwhelming to resist.

When the two women finally embraced, Barbara, who'd been laughing at her mother's outrageous antics a moment before, thought: *We'll be together again somehow.* She looked back from the terminal gate and caught the kiss Eileen blew, and then she moved towards the tunnel that led to the aircraft. She flew in silent withdrawal to San Francisco, where she'd catch the connecting flight to England, wondering when she'd see her mother again.

*It's a miracle! I'm cured!* It was fun in an airport lounge, light relief, but what Eileen needed was a *genuine* miracle, if she was going to be cured. She returned to the apartment, thinking how silent it would be now. There was the bed she'd shared with Barbara, the kitchen where they'd cooked together, the sofa where they'd sat talking: the emptiness was emphatic, resounding. She half-expected to hear Barbara's voice calling out – *want a cuppa tea, Mum? Anything I can get you to drink? You feeling OK?*

And then she noticed that Barbara had left behind a pair of shoes. She regarded this as a sign that her daughter would one day return.

*

On 20 October 1997, I received an e-mail from Barbara in Phoenix; it was my first communication from her. She wrote:

> *Dear Campbell, Hello! It is a wonderful experience to be part of this family. I feel as if I have known Stephen and Keiron for ever. The meeting with my Mum was the most amazing day of my life. The feeling between us is just as if we'd picked up from where we'd left off the last time we were together. I know that sounds strange, but it's the only way to describe it. It would be good to meet you sometime. Love, Barbara.*

I also received a note from Iain. *I met Barbara before she left*, he wrote. *I was wrong about her. She was extremely pleasant and helped Mom immensely.*

Early in November, after she'd returned to Yorkshire, Barbara wrote to her mother about what her time in Phoenix had meant: *I haven't truly processed those ten days we spent together. For now I want to say how wonderful it was for me. It was filled with very special moments . . . making tea for each other, folding the laundry, finding your socks, holding your hands, combing your hair, stroking your face while you slept, watching you sleep, eating chocolate, doing dishes, each of us looking for our glasses when they were on our heads, taking photos with the lens cover on, lying on the sofa with my head on your lap, singing* The Rose, *rubbing your back, massaging your feet, waking up to see you beside me . . . I will treasure every second I spent with you. Thank you for being my mum. I love you, Barbara.*

# 20

ON 4 November, Eileen checked into a retreat, run on holistic principles, that accepted cancer patients. It was operated by the clinic where she'd worked; ironically, she'd helped start this programme when she was healthy, and now she'd returned as a patient. On 18 November, she wrote to say that the experience had been 'good but gruelling'. She hadn't used oxygen or her wheelchair for the eleven days of the programme. She'd had massages and assorted physical therapy and special diets, and counselling sessions where she 'did some confrontation with her fear', which she found helpful. Now she was back at the apartment, and an unexpected depression she couldn't shift had settled on her.

She missed the protection and companionship of the programme; in the apartment she was on her own much of the time, experiencing what she called '*a constant battle between seeing improvements, and feeling lots of different things in my body which seem like disease progression*'. She wrote to me: '*Sometimes it's all such a long haul and not much to show for*

*it . . . then I have to remind myself of the trauma and onslaught
my body has experienced, and I'm grateful for how far I have
come.'*

How far *had* she come really? How far had she expected to
come? Her mood swung back and forth. She was making
progress, she wasn't making progress. She was inching forward, she was standing still. She didn't know what to believe,
what to think. Nancy Frick spent hours with her, and Iain
visited when he wasn't going to classes or burying himself in
textbooks, but the burden of looking after her fell largely on
Stephen, who was still sharing the apartment.

In the wretched circumstances of his mother's illness,
Stephen had blossomed. Before and during his marriage he'd
been unpunctual and unreliable, at times massively irrespon-
sible and self-destructive – in so many ways a mirror image of
my younger self, unmindful of clocks and obligations and
promises, clumsy with the feelings of others; now he was
always on time, or if he was delayed he'd telephone Eileen to
tell her so. He did the shopping, hauled out the garbage,
cooked, cleaned, did the laundry, made sure his mother was as
comfortable as she could be. He massaged her if she was in
pain, and when she was low he raised her up again – insisting
she could get through all this, she could come out of the darkness back into daylight, she could win. He was a source of
constant reassurance. *Get strong and well, Mother, you know
you can. Think positive thoughts.* These were scraps of her own
philosophy fed back to her; if you don't dwell on negative
thoughts, if you can free yourself of them, you can achieve
anything.

Stephen's was the therapy of quiet repetition and calm
patience with an infusion of humour too; he'd go through his
repertoire of mimicry and impressions – a 70s hippie on dope,
an Irishman who'd had too much Guinness, movie stars like

Woody Allen and Joe Pesci – or he'd come up with some absurd comic utterance or maybe a funny walk, and Eileen would laugh; but the stress of improvising to keep his mother afloat was beginning to wear on him.

He'd rise early, go to his job as a maintenance worker for a company that owned apartment complexes, then rush home again at the end of the day. At the same time he was exploring the possibility of putting his own family back together again, seeing his sons, discussing the future with his wife; but he realised that his marital life, coming undone as it might be, had to be put on hold because of his mother's illness. This took priority: Eileen's companion, helper, friend, confidant – it was a role he wanted, it satisfied him, redeemed him, strengthened his self-respect. He'd once said of his mother that 'she was proud of her kids, and she always wanted to be our best friend, and she definitely was'. This memory is one all the kids share, that of her friendship; and the fact that she was proud of them, she never discouraged them from their dreams or ambitions, no matter how far-fetched they might seem. *Go for it* was her philosophy. *Do it*. And if any of the boys had decisions to make, huge or small, she was there to discuss them. She was no conventional mother; she was too undomesticated, too unconcerned with the opinions of others, and sometimes a little too engrossed in her job at the clinic. She was often spacey, but she could also be eminently practical; like all of us, she embraced contradictions.

After our divorce, she'd thrown her home open to any of the kids' friends who had problems they wanted to talk about, stuff they couldn't discuss with their own parents. An open-house policy, and she never turned anyone away. And so kids would come around and they'd discuss life and all its myriad difficulties with her. She was a listener, a good one. It was almost as if she perceived the concept of motherhood as something that went beyond the needs of her own sons – it had an expandable quality.

Despite Stephen's attentions, and the phone calls that kept coming in from well-wishers and former colleagues and people who *still* wanted her to help analyse their dreams, Eileen was spending too much time on her own – there was loneliness as well as fear, long periods of silence and reflection and the sharp realisation that she wasn't improving. Quite the opposite. She was moving into a new stage of the disease. She was experiencing pain in parts of her body that had been pain-free zones before; there was more dread. The homeopathic remedies weren't helping; the alternative road to good health had been closed permanently. She was swallowing a dozen aspirins a day, or more.

She was in constant contact with Barbara. On 19 November she sent her an e-mail: *The pain in my shoulder is increasing and I am thinking of going to see an osteopath. Keep well in mind and spirit, much love as always, your mum.* Whether she saw the osteopath she never said. On 20 November she wrote again to Barbara: . . . *a couple of aspirin did the trick and I had a good night's sleep. I am reading some inspirational material before I fall asleep and when I wake. I must change my consciousness about this whole disease thing. I have so many memories of patients I've worked with who said 'if it wasn't for the pain I'd be able to cope'. I remember one woman crawling on the floor in agony one night and that haunts me still. I plan to make this a good day and wish the same for you, sweetie. Lots of love, your mum.*

A day later, I received an e-mail from Iain: *I am concerned about the increasing amounts of pain in her right shoulder. Frankly, I believe in drugs for their purposes – if you're in pain beyond aspirin, then get some Percodan. Why go through misery?*

Apart from the pain in her shoulder, a new and disturbing

symptom had appeared. Iain told me she'd developed a sore on the top of her head that had *gone from something small to something that looks like it should be in some dermatology journal. Dad, I don't like this situation and I wish it would go away and leave Mom to live the life she deserves to live.*

By late November she was taking aspirin every four hours. It didn't seem to have occurred to her that she should acquire a prescription painkiller, perhaps because she stubbornly didn't want to admit that the pain was out of control, or that she'd failed to check it with the power of 'positive thinking', or that the homeopathic remedies – in which she'd put such so much faith – hadn't helped bring her relief. When Iain suggested Percodan, she dismissed the idea.

On 22 November, she told Barbara that she was worried about her shoulder: *It's a bit scary, Barbara. I don't have much faith in doctors or perhaps it is just that they do not think they can do anything for me now. I spend a lot of time in prayer, praying for the right action, and of course for healing for you and me. I wish I could make it all better.*

A couple of days later Eileen sent another note: *Barbara: you are such a strength for me. I know God planned this, you coming into my life and me into yours, at this time. I am so glad you are in my life. I do not know how I can tell you how much you mean to me. Not only for who you are, and the magnificent being you are, but you have become a good friend and you can make me laugh in the most joyous way. I miss you so much. Stay well, my love, your mum.*

Iain, meantime, had written to tell me that Eileen was going to see a dermatologist about the sore on top of her head. He added: *Nancy and Mom's physician friends have the feeling that her condition is worsening and that her cancer has probably spread. Nancy suggests that I begin preparing myself for the worst. I love Mom so much and I don't and won't give up hope at this time.* Perhaps echoing his mother unconsciously, he added: *We need to be extremely positive, now more than ever.*

I replied to him on 25 November, saying how powerless I felt in the situation. *I think in my head I am preparing for the worst, but in my heart I am saying No, something good has to happen . . . What we do in a situation like this is hope and encourage.*

How empty my words seemed, like a voice whispering in a gale. What a poor cheerleader I made.

I was in Ireland, working on a book; it was half-hearted labour. *Preparing for the worst.* But you can never really prepare. It's not as if you can go into training for grief, doing exercises on a daily basis. What regime would you follow – crying into a handkerchief? Looking gloomy? Trying on funereal clothes? It's a bullshit idea that you can prepare yourself for the worst; you're *never* ready.

I knew Eileen was dying, but I'd tried to shove the idea to the back of my head and get on with my life, because I didn't want to picture her slipping deathwards, not Eileen, not the mother of our kids, the source of so many memories, times of happiness, sadness, times after the end of the marriage when we didn't communicate with regularity even if there were things we may have wanted to say to each other. We assumed, as humans often do, that somehow we're imperishable, we have a licence to procrastinate, and we think yeah, well, one day we'll get around to talking at length, and you can tell me how you are and if life is being kind to you, and if you've discovered a satisfactory relationship with somebody – but such conversations didn't happen with any kind of consistency. And now I wished they had. This saddened me. Too much had been postponed, then forgotten or lost.

So in Ireland, in my cluttered room overlooking dismal

rainy fields and a sodden low-clouded scowling sky, I smoked scores of cigarettes and picked at the fabric of the book, I revised more than I created, I shuffled sentences and paragraphs around, I found myself staring at the same sentence time and again, buffing it, reworking it, then putting it back the way it had been before I tampered with it. I was disengaged from this fiction; I wasn't in Ireland in spirit. I knew it was only a matter of time before I'd go back to Arizona.

Sometimes I took the car and drove backroads to escape the confines of my office and the seemingly pointless demands of my work. I'd go through villages and see turf-smoke, spreading its vaguely marijuana-like perfume, rise towards a frosty moon, and lights glow in the windows of pubs. How tempting it was to park the car and go inside one of the bars and hoist myself up on a worn leather stool at the counter and ask for a pint of Guinness and lose myself in drink and smoke and the idle chitchat of an Irish country pub.

How simple all that seemed, the old escape route of booze, the tunnel that led you into that place where nobody dies any death other than one that is noble and dignified. But I didn't want to drink. I wanted what I couldn't have: Eileen's well-being.

Her life.

I phoned her one day in November. There were pauses between her words, little vacuums. The substance of our conversation I've largely forgotten; I remember telling her I was planning to visit again, I just wasn't sure when. I asked to speak to Stephen. She told me he'd just stepped outside, he had an errand to run; then she said, 'Wait,' and I heard a sound of her moving. Minutes later, she came back on the line.

'Christ,' she said, and her accent was pure Glasgow. She was gasping for air. 'That was a first. I just ran after him. I haven't run anywhere in a long time.' She may have been trying to laugh at her own physical inadequacy; I like to think that's what the wheezing sound suggested. She was looking for humour at the heart of her misery.

Stephen took over the phone. I told him I was planning to visit, but it probably wouldn't be until just after Christmas – I had a book to deliver and the funds due would help finance the trip; at the back of my mind was the cold prospect that there might not be an 'after Christmas' for Eileen. *Don't die yet, Eileen. Hang in. Even if there's nothing I can do for you, I'm coming.* Stephen was happy I'd be making the trip. He told me that Sydney was due to arrive from Glasgow shortly; and that Barbara was arranging a second visit.

In Yorkshire, all the fizz and euphoria Barbara had brought back with her from the United States was beginning to disintegrate in the face of the fact that her mother's condition was worsening at a frightening pace. It was easier to tell from the phone calls than the e-mails that Eileen was suffering. Her voice was distant to the point that she sounded as if she were in a trance; she might try to disguise it, but she couldn't conceal from Barbara her despair and deterioration.

Nancy Frick had taken Eileen for an X-ray of the shoulder, but the results had come back as inconclusive, a word that has always seemed to me like doctorspeak for ignorance.

A bone scan was recommended but Eileen was becoming exhausted by pain, and spending most of her time in bed now, and so the notion of the scan was allowed to slip away unfulfilled. The dermatologist removed the growth from Eileen's scalp; whether it was cancerous or not, I never learned. Her illness was spinning out of control by this time anyway – new bumps, lumps, aches, pains; and mentally she was sinking into a mire of alienation and despondency.

Barbara wrote in her journal that she was longing to go to her mother and take care of her, an urge that increased with each phone call. Once, Eileen phoned to say she needed to take a bath, but wasn't sure if she'd be able to manage it without help, because of her pain (and she was probably too embarrassed to ask Stephen for assistance). This was *the* crux for Barbara, the turning point where she decided she'd go back, no matter what it took. She didn't mention the decision to Eileen, in case for some reason she *couldn't* make it to Arizona. She knew her mother needed her – not just as a daughter, but also as a nurse.

There was the question of raising money for the fare, and the prospect of making the long trip alone, but when Barbara was determined to achieve something – as she'd done when she'd doggedly hunted the faint crisscrossing tracks left down the years by her mother – she usually managed to succeed. The bank refused her a loan. She was unemployed now, a bad risk. She turned to generous relatives, who gave her the money without question. Elated, Barbara booked the first flight to Phoenix she could find – Nick understood she had to go, no power on earth or elsewhere could have stopped her when it came to her mother – and then she phoned Eileen.

After some general chat, Barbara asked the question she'd been saving as a big surprise. 'How would you like a nice bed bath from your daughter?'

Eileen said, 'Oh God, a bed bath would be wonderful—'

'You think you can wait until Sunday?' Barbara asked.

'Sunday?' Eileen sounded confused.

'Sunday,' Barbara said. 'I'll be there around four o'clock. I need my shoes back, Mum.'

Eileen realised: *her daughter was coming back to her*. She sobbed tears of excitement and anticipation; this was a wild fantasy turning real. *Barbara would arrive and make her strong*

*again, Barbara could take the pain away. She needed Barbara.*
She hadn't dared to hope she'd ever see her daughter again –
not in this lifetime.

Barbara felt enough confidence to make the trip unaccom-
panied. She'd had the results of the scan that was done before
her first trip to Arizona, and the tumours had diminished –
there was reduction of the infected areas in chest glands, and
both lungs showed clear areas apart from a few small nodules.
The mass on the colon had completely disappeared.

She was looking better too. Her hair was growing back, the
circles under her eyes were gone, the colour was returning to
her face. She had begun to resemble her old self.

On 30 November she left Yorkshire to make the trip to
Arizona. Her flight seemed longer than her first journey. The
mood this time was different, sombre. This was no joyful
reunion. There would be no parties, no fun outings to scenic
spots. She was going to a place where there were no coloured
balloons and buffets and awesome Red Rock landscapes.
Stephen, relieved to see his sister again, met her at Sky Harbor
Airport and drove her to the apartment. He'd changed; he
was grim and troubled, uncertain about the future, his own
and his mother's.

Eileen was in bed, face shrunken, wasting. She was in great
pain, the worst so far: the fiery intensity of it racked her. She
was burning up, fevered. Barbara spent that long dreadful
insomniac Sunday night trying to console and comfort her
mother, but the pain was too extreme for words and gestures
of solace to alleviate. This was a place way beyond the reaches
of aspirin, beyond codeine. First thing in the morning, she
contacted the local Hospice, and within hours nurses arrived
and morphine was administered. A social worker also called to
explain the full range of Hospice services – counselling,

ministerial visits, oxygen equipment, whatever would ease the patient's concerns.

Apart from the morphine in tablet form, Eileen was allowed a liquid version, Roxinall, to be used for 'break-through' pain, which was happening frequently. Barbara developed a relaxation routine for her mother, massaging her feet and legs, during which time Eileen kept repeating *I am strong, I am in control, I am calm.* The comfort of affirmations. The lulling effect of repetitions. The same chant over and over, same song, self-hypnosis. These sessions happened regularly at night; Eileen rarely slept for more than a couple of hours at any time, so Barbara could only catnap, waking when her mother stirred, to begin the sessions again. Or to bathe Eileen, change her clothes, brush her hair.

Although the morphine brought Eileen the first real relief she'd felt in a long time, it also made her listless, stoned, easily confused. Iain wrote me to say that he wished she didn't have to take the stuff, he didn't like how her eyes became droopy and her habit of falling asleep in mid-conversation – but when he weighed these disadvantages against the severity of pain, it was no contest. He also expressed his concern that morphine would take the fight out of her, she wouldn't have the will to combat cancer any more. He was still living in unscientific hope, dreaming of some ultimate victory, or the faint possibility of one. He added that it was comforting to have Barbara back.

She had a way of spreading reassurance around, of easing into control of a situation without dominating it. There was nothing domineering in her manner. Only a truly charitable soul could have the capacity to ignore her own cancer and care for someone else's. And even if her disease had stalled for the present, she knew it could rear up again just like *that*, it was volatile and sneaky, and ruthless in the violence it might wreak on the human body.

She had only to look at her mother's face to see that cancer devastated with all the force of an uncontrollable forest fire.

I asked Nancy Frick about the timing of my proposed visit; I was putting her on the spot. The implied question was: how long has Eileen got? And that was unanswerable. Nancy wrote back on 4 December: *Things are not predictable here. I wish I knew what to tell you about your plans to come over. I can tell you that Eileen is deteriorating. She's not eating enough, she's getting thinner and weaker . . . I'll help answer any questions you have, but I don't know about the most important one: How long do we have? Don't be sad. She and Iain and Stephen and Keiron (still in Seattle) have had talks, and they have all come to accept that she may not be staying here.*

Nancy's last phrase wrung my heart out of shape.

Sydney arrived a few days after Barbara. Effectively, he'd come to say goodbye to his sister, although he would never have uttered this aloud to anyone, and may not even have admitted it to himself. He loved her, and she him; they were opposites, they'd spent most of their lives apart. Eileen had always been the more adventurous, impulsive, fun-loving; Sydney was conservative, set in his ways, didn't like to act without thinking through the consequences. Eileen had moved from Glasgow to London to New York, and then westward to Arizona; Sydney had always remained in the small, known world of Glasgow. She'd more or less rejected her Jewishness; Sydney adhered to his.

He came carrying a suitcase generously stuffed with Scottish gifts for her, items difficult to locate in Arizona; traditional Scottish butter shortbread, Scottish candies (*sweeties* in Glaswegian parlance: there is nothing so blood-numbingly sweet and viciously tooth-rotting as Edinburgh Rock or McCowan's Highland Toffee, wondrously vile, the bane and yet the prosperity of dentists from Stranraer to Skye), tea towels depicting Highland scenes, scarves, clothing from Marks & Spencer.

Barbara hadn't met him face to face before; there had been the tense seven weeks of phone conversations in the summer, the delayed letter, the weekend health updates, but no physical encounter until now. She felt a little nervous, wondered if he had any bad feelings towards her, if there was resentment over the fact that she'd forced his hand about making contact with Eileen. But Sydney was pleased to meet her, even if his attention was less focused on Barbara than on the health of his sister, whose appearance distressed him.

He'd expected her to look ill – but not this, not this declining, spindly woman who was in and out of morphine sleep, and who'd been administered a dose shortly before his arrival. She cried quietly when she saw him. It must have reached her through the gauze of the drug that her brother hadn't travelled all the way from Scotland for a vacation; he'd come because she was very sick, because this might be their last meeting, she was straddling worlds, dark and light – she must have recognised this, seen it in his expression and his manner, which was solicitous and kindly. Did she think, *I'm dying and Sid's here because we may never meet again?*

I wonder how it feels to look at somebody, even through the fog of morphine, and realise that the time left to you is seriously limited – does the drug dull the dread as much as it stifles the pain? Does it twist reality enough so that you don't have an inkling that you're close to the last exit? Or do you sense around you strands of mist gathering? Whatever was going through her mind, Eileen was happy Sydney had come; he was family, the last connection with her dead parents, he brought an air of dear old faraway Glasgow with him, and it was good to hear the familiar accent again.

Barbara and Sydney got along with no uneasiness. They shared a serious common concern. At nights, sometimes, when Eileen was sleeping, Sydney would talk in a whisper, like a man in a library, about his fear that his sister might die while he was in Phoenix and that would mean a funeral, and he wasn't sure he could cope with one; or he'd thank Barbara for looking after Eileen, because he'd never have been able to do what she was doing. He didn't have the heart for it.

He slept in Stephen's sofa bed, and Stephen moved out to stay with friends for the duration of Sydney's visit. (For Stephen, this was a welcome interlude, a break from strain.) During the day, Sydney liked to go out for bagels and smoked salmon, and he'd bring them back to tempt Eileen into eating them, but her appetite was poor, and she wasn't interested very often.

In her times of clarity, Eileen went through severe emotional dips. She was sick of the dismal, deteriorating quality of her life, weary of medication and her inability to motivate herself, tired of her lack of mobility – and who could blame her? During these periods, Barbara would try to jog her into having a better attitude – but that familiar old problem rears up yet again: *what can you say?* Once, Barbara told her that they hadn't been given this disease to deal with on their own, they'd been given it to deal with together at the same time, for some reason. Unity of purpose, fight back in tandem. They were a team. Maybe that was why they'd been reunited at this particular time: to kill off the disease.

'We can't do it alone,' Barbara said. 'It's too big for either one of us to do it singly, we have to join forces, join power. You pull me back in, I pull you back in . . .'

Eileen said, 'And no matter what the doctors tell us, that our situations aren't hopeful – that doesn't make any sense to me.'

They lay on the bed, holding each other, Barbara trying to infuse her mother with some of her own strength, which wasn't infinite. And once, when Barbara had a lapse into sadness and cried, Eileen placed Barbara's head on her breast and patted it and said, 'I know, darling, I know. The past is the past, and all we have is now . . . it doesn't feel right that we found each other just to die. It doesn't make sense.'

Let me do it, let me impose sense, it's what I try to do, it's what I can't help trying—

*They rise from the bed together. They walk out into the sunlight. Eileen has an arm linked through Barbara's. They feel warmth on their faces. They stroll around the swimming pool where a few dead leaves are whipped toward the drain by the snakelike device that cleans the water. They sit down at one of the tables and watch sun in the blue pool and how the surface of water changes shape and sparkles.*

*Eileen says, 'Look,' and points to an object half-hidden by the leaves of a yucca plant. 'It's hard to believe I needed that, isn't it?'*

*Barbara laughs. 'There was a time you couldn't get anywhere without it, Mum.'*

*'It's rusted, look at it.'*

*'You don't need it now,' Barbara says. 'Let it rust. Who cares.'*

*She reaches for her mother's hand across the table. Their fingers touch. Eileen's skin is cool. A bluejay flies up from the yucca behind which the old wheelchair is half-hidden. Eileen looks at the familiar object. Spokes are broken and twisted; leather upholstery has cracked in the heat and discoloured stuffing material sticks out; the tyres are flat and the chrome surfaces turned to brown. She turns away from the sight, gazes at Barbara.*

*'You look good,' Eileen says.*

*'I feel good,' Barbara answers.*

*'We did it, didn't we?'*

*'We did it. You're right.'*

*'Damn right,'* Eileen says.

*'We beat it, Mum.'*

*'Together.'*

*'We were united against it—'*

*'And we won, they said we couldn't do it, but we did, God we really did.'*

*'Together,'* Barbara says.

*She pulls her hand away to swat at a fly that has landed on her arm—*

But I can't make it work, I can't get this fiction to hang together, the images are gauzy, and the two women seem to be receding inside a mist I can't disperse, they're fading, and I don't have the power to bring them back into focus, I try, I try, but it's slipping beyond my reach, even as I grope for it.

Occasionally Eileen was able to correspond with me by e-mail. She tried to make fun of her condition. In early December she wrote: *Hi Campbell, If I told you there's a lot of bridge under the water, would you say this was a confused person? . . . This gives you an idea of what it is like with me and my medications. I laugh at myself sometimes. I start sentences and don't know where they're going. I drift. Last night I found myself reaching for my cigarette before I realised I hadn't smoked in eight years. Barbara's visit has been incredible. I forget she has her own physical challenges and she does so much for me . . . The Hospice people come directly to the house, they know more about pain management than any of the doctors. I know that 'hospice' gives the connotation of 'the end of the road', but Barbara put me straight on that, helping me to see it as the beginning of pain management and being able to function on a better level . . . It is*

*at times like this that cancer doesn't seem to have much room in
my life.*

The end of Barbara's visit was approaching; again, she
faced the prospect of leaving her mother. She made a list of
instructions for the other helpers to use after she'd gone, a
daily programme of medications, passive exercises, and relaxation sessions. She knew Stephen would do his best, and that
Nancy was a constant visitor, and the Hospice staff were
always on call. She was running on empty after the demands of
her stay, and distraught about leaving. What else could she do?
Christmas was coming. The festive season, gifts to be bought,
a tree to dress, a family waiting for her. And, for her family's
sake, she had to make an effort at normality, even as she wondered what it would have been like to spend one Christmas –
*one single goddamn Christmas out of forty-two wasn't much to
ask, was it?* – with her mother. She wanted to cook Christmas
dinner for her, pull a Christmas cracker with her, and sit down
to a meal of turkey and cranberry sauce. But she was to be
robbed of all this, just as she'd been cheated of too many years
of her mother's life. She kept telling herself: be bloody grateful for what you have. She might never have met her mother at
all, and that would have been worse, but at least they'd met,
they'd got to know each other, and they'd loved, how they'd
loved.

On the morning of her departure, 14 December, Barbara
was reluctant to go. Eileen told her, 'I don't want your leaving
to be a big thing. We just have to do it with as little fuss as possible. OK?'

Barbara said OK. Her suitcases were already packed. All
she had to do was step out the door, Stephen would take her to
the airport, that was it. She hugged her mother. Both women
were well aware, as Barbara put it, that they'd stolen even
more precious time together, and couldn't dare to hope they'd

ever meet again. This was it, the end of it: as she walked out of the apartment she thought, *I've seen my mother for the last time.*

She returned to Yorkshire. She felt a great winter inside, a grief deep as a pit. There were absences in her world. She wrote: *Although I have found my long-lost mother, I'm soon to be motherless again . . . Why?*

Sydney left four days after Barbara. A few days before his departure, he brushed Eileen's hair for her, probably for the first time ever. It wasn't a masculine thing, it was something women did for each other. Eileen was moved by the gesture because she knew it made her brother feel a little awkward; Sydney worked the brush in short strokes, trying to be gentle, careful of her scalp and the place where she'd had surgery done. Brother and sister together, and the drone of the oxygen concentrator in the background, and lamplight reflected palely in the plastic oxygen tube attached to Eileen's nostrils. Sydney knew one thing for certain as he drew the brush up and down: it was the first time he'd ever done this, and it would also be the last.

Barbara telephoned Eileen frequently. Often Eileen was too short of breath to speak or too heavily medicated to come to the phone. A couple of catchphrases were developed to camouflage the difficulty of communication. Barbara would always ask, 'Is this my wee Mum?'

And Eileen would always answer: 'This is your wee Mum. Is this my daughter?'

It was the best Eileen could do, and her decline was breaking Barbara's heart, already strained to the limit and beyond.

# 21

A week before Christmas, I booked tickets for Rebecca and myself on a flight from Dublin to Phoenix, departing 10 January. I'd tried to get an earlier flight, but nothing was available. Our plan was to stay in Arizona for two weeks. I wasn't thinking in terms of saying goodbye to Eileen. That lay in some nebulous future and, cowardly, I didn't want to look ahead in any case.

On 24 December Stephen wrote to me: *Hey Dad, How's it going? Pretty good here. Just wrapping up Christmas presents and watching Mom eat a little waffle and eggs. I can't wait to see you. My love to you and Rebecca.*

The waffle and eggs Stephen mentioned would have amounted to no more than three or four bites. Eileen's appetite was a source of serious concern now. She wasn't interested in eating. The combination of morphine and cancer was killing her desire for food, and she was inevitably growing weaker. Nancy Frick had written to me about this, adding that a day would come – very soon, she felt – when Eileen would have to be moved to a facility where she could be looked after properly, and fed intravenously. The idea of Eileen living in such a place saddened and appalled Nancy, but Stephen couldn't take care of his mother full-time. Nor could Nancy, who was busy looking for a new job. The Hospice people were generous at times to the point of sainthood, but they didn't have the staff to provide a nurse round the clock.

I wasn't sure what I could do to help in this situation; I'd be flying, as I'd done the previous summer, into the unknown. But it was a different unknown now, because the variables had become fixed and defined: last time at least there had been laser surgery and radiation therapy, and a chance of tumours shrinking and maybe God smiling down from Up Above in benevolent mode, but this time there were no surgical protocols left, only fragile ungrounded human hope. Maybe she'll improve. Maybe she'll have one of those totally puzzling, almost mythical, remissions. It was a hope so faint it had less resonance than a frail harp-string plucked gently in a room far away and vibrating only a few shivering seconds. After that there was silence and the hard indigestible gristle of truth: she was dying, she'd been dying since last July. And long before that.


In Yorkshire, Barbara went through the motions of the festive season. She brooded over her mother's sickness. In a time of tinsel and gifts and plastic angels parked on Christmas trees and glitter dangling from branches, the quintessential family time, she tried to resign herself to the idea that she'd seen Eileen for the last time. When she telephoned her mother on New Year's Eve, she was struck by how weak Eileen's voice had become, how fast her health was failing. Barbara reflected sorrowfully on the fact that this was the first time in her life she'd ever been able to wish her real mother Happy New Year: but how much of 1998 would Eileen live to see? *I wonder if I'll ever be able to*

*hold her in my arms again,* Barbara wrote, *or if I'll see her smile.*
She was beginning to grieve, to accept the idea that she and her
mother would never be together again.

Phone conversations were strictly limited now by Eileen's
strength or mental acuity, little ordeals that Barbara would go
through; she wished she could be in her mother's room again,
lying beside her, helping her even as she moved into that ill-lit
uncharted hinterland beyond help. Just being there for her –
that was all Barbara wanted now.

She was also being realistic, and knew that between her and
her mother they couldn't overwhelm the cancer, no matter how
many affirmations they made together, no matter how positive
and powerful they might imagine they felt in combination. All
the self-help mantras in the world, the strange potions and
putative cures – these had been vanquished by the disease. At
the end of every phone call, Barbara wondered if that was to be
the last contact she'd have with Eileen. Would there be another
call? And another after that? It was all sadness and uncertainty.
*The long search ends,* Barbara wrote, *in a place where I can never
find her this time.*

Nancy phoned with the news that Eileen was getting confused more frequently. On several occasions she'd imagined
that Barbara was at the airport in Phoenix, waiting to be picked
up and brought to her. Increasingly, Eileen had been asking:
'Where is Barbara? Where is she? Isn't she coming?'

Her family knew the strain Barbara was under; they understood her sorrow and how powerless she felt. They also realised
too the division in her life, that she lived half in Yorkshire, half
in Arizona. And who could live in two places simultaneously
without sooner or later coming unstitched?

Iain and Stephen met Rebecca and me at the airport in Phoenix
on 10 January. We were tired; it was too late to visit Eileen, who

wasn't expecting us until morning in any case. We ate Mexican food with the boys in a boisterous restaurant a mile or so from the airport. We were joined by Rebecca's mother and stepfather – they live in Phoenix – and a couple of Stephen's kids, Neal and Connor, one of whom was sleepy, the other hyperactive.

I felt light-headed, unfocused, the aeroplane still zoomed in my skull. The mess of food on my plate looked like splashes of spilled acrylic paint, a psychedelic effect, and the conversation around the table was fractured and almost inaudible against the noisy background. I went outside to the parking lot to smoke. Stephen followed me. The air smelled of gasoline fumes and fried onions and peppers. 10 January and warm, and a city moon the colour of an old penny in the sky. It was strange to be back in Phoenix.

We smoked in silence for a while. I watched him, wondered what was going on inside his mind. Wondered how he'd managed to stay intact under the weight of caring for his mother. Or if he'd broken in places I couldn't see. How did he juggle the different demands of his life? Wife and kids, Eileen, the long hours he worked?

'How are you holding up?' I asked.

'I'm OK, Dad. I worry about her when I'm not with her during the day,' he said.

'I'll help,' I said. I wasn't sure how, in a practical sense, to take some of the load from Stephen, tote a little of that weight he'd been carrying. 'Rebecca will help as well. That's why we're here.'

'It's great you've come,' he said. '. . . Mom doesn't know what's going on a lot of the time. But she'll get a lift out of seeing you.'

Something was burning inside the restaurant kitchen, oil maybe, jalapenos flaming in grease. The smell floated towards us. I regarded the lit end of my cigarette. 'This crap,' and I

shook my head, disgusted that seven months had passed since
Stephen and I had smoked together, and I was *still* hooked on
the absurd habit. 'Fuck this,' I said. I dropped the cigarette and
crushed it with my foot and went back inside the restaurant.

The hotel we checked into was one of those efficiency places
with a kitchen, newly constructed and devoid of character, a
concrete box on the edge of the freeway. It was utilitarian, but
we hadn't come here for a luxury vacation. This was no sight-
seeing jaunt through the great Southwest.

That first night I thought I'd sleep forever. Rebecca was
weary too, but in the event we slept only an infuriatingly short
time, waking at six AM and then driving – in the Buick we'd borrowed from her mother – to a twenty-four-hour supermarket,
so vast and so empty and so fluorescent that it suggested a
structure left intact, by some freak chance, after a nuclear holo-
caust. Where was the population – pulverised by the blast?
Phoenix had always seemed temporary to me anyway, a transient city the desert would ultimately reclaim. I imagined
abandoned buildings, paint burned off windowframes and
doors by the climate, deserted cars blistered by the sun, a great
hot emptiness and tumbleweed rolling slowly along cracked
pavement where weeds sprouted. And all the shopping malls
and plazas were filled with fine grit blown in from the Saguaro
Desert, and dust-clogged traffic signals flickered intermittently
then crackled and died. And the city was gone.

We rolled our cart along wide vacant aisles, remembering
stuff we hadn't seen since we'd moved to Ireland – Dr Pepper
and Kraft Macaroni & Cheese in packets and Dolly Madison
ice cream. Stuff and more stuff. I wondered how much imagination and energy went into, say, the invention of yet another
breakfast cereal – dear Christ, how much choice did people
really *need*? How many ways can you tart up a cornflake?

We bought a few essential provisions, and then I stopped where I knew I'd been headed all along – the pharmacy section: this was the Moment of Decision. The road junction where your life changes.

This way or that. Which route to take?

I made up a brief list of what I thought I'd be losing – the luxury of the after-dinner cigarette, arguably the finest smoke of the day; the cigarette that goes along with your coffee; the smokes you light without thinking when you sit down to tap at your keyboard; the cigarette you need when you're on the telephone . . . Goddammit, do it, just do the thing, this shillyshallying was nonsense; I picked up a box of nicotine patches and tossed them inside the shopping cart and I thought of Eileen and lung cancer and dying, and I realised I had to give these patches a chance, I'd take a shot at them, the pangs of withdrawal surely couldn't last for long, and in any event they were nothing, they were *minuscule*, insignificant *itches*, compared to the agonies of cancer.

Back at the hotel, I opened one of the patches and stuck it on my upper arm. There was a smell – vaguely medicinal but reminiscent of nothing I'd encountered before. I imagined nicotine being released into my bloodstream. I thought of the captain of my cortex, enslaved by tobacco, waiting for his first sweet hit of the morning; and I wondered if the patch would deceive him, or if he'd be so enraged by the trickery he'd redirect my brain and – like a madman intent on ramming his ferryboat into a riverbank – command me to smoke a real cigarette at once. Would I capsize and be lost? Would I sink to the bottom of the river of good intentions, the deranged captain staring at me with hatred even as he also drowned?

Rebecca said, 'You might not have picked the best time to quit. Good luck.'

I tapped the patch, pressing it harder against my flesh. I thought that if I applied pressure, nicotine would be released all the more quickly. Thus do we addicts deceive ourselves, looking for tricks and shortcuts, even when we're attempting to conquer our addictions.

We drove to the apartment. Stephen, who'd been expecting us, opened the patio door. Eileen was sitting on the sofa in the living room, awaiting our arrival. She smiled when she saw us. I took her hand and sat alongside her. I'd been prepared for changes in her appearance, but she was diminished beyond my expectations. She looked hollow; she might have been possessed by a malicious spirit draining her from within. Her colour was poor, as if no blood ran in her veins. There was an element of baffled anxiety about her too – the way she fidgeted with her oxygen tube, which she sometimes took from her nostrils and looked at, as if puzzled by the purpose of such a thing. She lacked concentration. Her voice was lifeless. I asked her some inconsequential question – something to do with the medication she was taking, I don't remember now – and she answered, 'I don't want to talk about my health.'

In fact, she didn't want to talk about anything. She was holding Rebecca's hand also now. 'I'm sorry, I'm tired,' she said, in that distant whisper of hers that seemed to accentuate her Scots accent. 'Don't think I'm rude. I need to rest.'

'You're not being rude,' I said.

I led her inside the bedroom, where a miniature Christmas tree with red and pink lights burned on a bookshelf; I found this little leftover festive touch upsetting. I had an abrupt flash of Christmases past when we'd been together and the kids had been young and Eileen healthy, and how there had always been that early Christmas morning ritual – practically pagan in its intensity – when the kids rose in unison, as if orchestrated the night before by big brother Iain, and attacked the wrapped gifts Santa had left under the tree. And then they'd come inside our bedroom, scattering their bounty around, bouncing on the bed, *look what Santa brought us*! When Iain and Stephen were non-believers in Father Christmas, they kept up the illusion for the sake of Keiron. Sad to remember all that, like bringing back an old used-up life, a place you'd never go again. A dead past, beyond salvage – yet trapped inside the brain, held there by the rusting girders of memory.

The oxygen concentrator rattled against the wall. On the circular bedside table were pills, crumpled tissues, cottonbuds, a glass of water with tiny bubbles adhering to the inside, a lamp.

I helped Eileen lie down. She said, 'I want to talk to Rebecca later. In private.' And then she shut her eyes.

This was to become a pattern, this desire to set time aside for Rebecca. And I knew Rebecca wanted that too. She'd always felt she and Eileen would have become friends if geography hadn't intervened. There was no animosity between them, an unusual condition to exist between a man's former wife and his present one. But it had happened that way. On Keiron's graduation from high school, Eileen had even written Rebecca a warm letter thanking her for helping bring Keiron up. In turn, Eileen had unreservedly welcomed Leda into her family, looked forward to her company at Sunday afternoon barbecues, came to care for her.

I couldn't relate this woman, this shell of a person, to my ex-wife, who'd been vibrant, energetic, smart, a little whacky. I remembered the accurate and funny way Stephen had once described her: *down to earth and out to lunch*. I sat beside the bed until she was asleep. I knew in that moment, with the oxygen machine churning and the laboured sound of Eileen's breathing and the way she held the transparent plastic tube slackly between her long thin fingers, I wouldn't leave Phoenix until it was all over, one way or another.

And there could only be one way. I couldn't keep the dented ping-pong ball of optimism in the air any longer.

The subject of putting Eileen into an institution was raised again, this time by one of the Hospice nurses, but the family – Iain, Stephen and myself (Keiron was in Seattle and yet to arrive) – rejected the idea without debate. It might have made our lives easier and more convenient to have somebody care for her, but *dammit*, this was a human being we all loved, this was the mother of our three sons, this woman had been my wife once, no way was she going inside some kind of home for the terminally ill where she'd be fed through tubes, no way was she going to spend what little time remained of her life among strangers, lying doped in a ward and left to drift out of this world with nobody around her she knew or recognised. What if, dying, she raised a hand at the last to search for somebody familiar, to touch the face of somebody she loved, what if she had a moment of penetrating clarity and wanted some comforting contact in the last few moments of her life – and there was nobody nearby? We all die alone; but we don't have to die in alien circumstances, in a strange place with fresh-laundered white sheets suggestive of shrouds against our flesh, and some distant nurse nasally announcing a message for Dr So and So through a loudspeaker system, and orderlies coming and going along corridors with gurneys and portable X-ray machines and oxygen equipment: what if all this was her very last outburst of perception, this glacial activity going on all around, and none of it had anything to do with her life and death? She'd have nobody to say goodbye to. Nobody to look at for the last time. She'd be utterly alone.

She needed full-time assistance, fine, OK, somehow we'd do it ourselves, it required only a little organisation and patience. We quickly set up our own shift-system of care. Nancy Frick and I agreed we'd do the morning and afternoon watches together; Nancy would come to the apartment around seven, when Stephen had to leave for work, and I'd join her between nine-thirty and ten. Rebecca would relieve one or other of us now and again, and Stephen take over when he came home from work. Iain was responsible for assuming Stephen's role on some nights. At other times Iain's girlfriend Juleah, a student from Yuma, would spend several hours on duty: Juleah was a surprise, a bolt from the blue; typically, he'd never mentioned her to me. His life was like a black velvet bag with a drawstring he sometimes tugged to open, and he'd sparingly spill a surprise. Here, this is a privileged glimpse into my world. Look quick before I pull the bag shut.

We circulated as best we could, according to our energies and obligations elsewhere. On certain nights Rebecca's contribution was to take Stephen out and make sure he relaxed over a few drinks. It was important that he spend as much time away from the apartment as we could arrange: he'd put in his hours, and more. We worked to no rigid timetable, we didn't punch time-clocks, the set-up was entirely flexible. We had only one rule: Eileen was never to be left on her own.

How practical we became, how adept at administering her medications, the liquid morphine, the cough medication, the tranquillisers, the laxatives, the morphine in tab form – all the capsules that kept her functioning. It was my first experience of the common humanity that comes to the fore in the face of death, a bonding of people, as if what we're really looking at in a dying person's eyes is our own inescapable future; the mortality, not of one person, but of the species.

I was awed by the generosity and concern of others. It

wasn't just Nancy and the hours she spent lying on the bed beside Eileen and whispering to her in a reassuring way or laughing with her or reminiscing about the years they'd worked at the clinic, it wasn't only Stephen's steadfast patience and Iain's constant concern with his mother's breathing and the way he'd make sure the oxygen supply was correct or how he'd apply a suction tube to her windpipe (he'd done this hundreds of times as a respiratory therapist), it wasn't the surprising reservoir of endurance I discovered in myself, and it wasn't the supercharged kindness of Hospice nurses and aides who came and went, it was also the endless phone calls from Eileen's friends and colleagues and those she'd helped at the clinic, calls she was rarely able to answer herself. I sometimes took them on her behalf. *Tell her we're praying for her. Tell her we're thinking of her constantly.*

I knew she'd given most of her life over to helping others through the medium of the clinic, but I'd had no real idea of the extent of her giving, nor the esteem in which she was held. She wasn't perfect. Nobody is. But she was a good person, and her heart was that rare chamber – a cave filled with the treasure of kind intentions.

Good people, in this unjust world of ours, often die bad deaths.

She still had the occasional desire to get out in her wheelchair. Nancy or Stephen or I would push her around the apartment complex, and she'd sit by the edge of the swimming pool. She rarely spoke. Often she wanted to know the time, and when you told her she always looked surprised; it didn't matter how you answered her question – two-thirty, four o'clock – she'd raise her eyebrows as if to say *Already? Where has the day flown?* Or maybe she was asking: *Where have all the years gone? Is this the end, is this all there is to life?*

At times she seemed, with her head tipped to the side, to be listening for something – birdsong, an aeroplane overhead, or a thing more profound and mysterious and ethereal, I could never tell, never guess. She spent ages fidgeting with her oxygen tube, checking the attachment to her nostrils as if she suspected a blockage was hindering the flow of oxygen to her lungs; but there was never any impediment in the long plastic line.

She'd begun to live increasingly in a world shaped by morphine, a place of shadow with only a fragile connection to reality. She developed the suspicion that she wasn't getting the correct number of pills – she was taking too many, she wasn't taking enough, she shouldn't be taking any at all. On scores of occasions, we had to explain the function of each item of medication; somebody would place a capsule in the palm of her hand and say, 'This brown tab is the laxative, Eileen.' And then: 'This little white tab is the Lorazepam for anxiety. The small blue one is the morphine.' Time and again, this was the procedure.

She'd take one of the pills into her mouth and spit it out with a look in her eye of grave doubt. She developed a special dislike for the liquid morphine, which was used to control break-through pain. She refused to take it. Iain and I decided to add few drops of the drug to her drinking water, and see if she noticed. At first, she sipped the water, and said nothing; some time later, in a brief moment of clarity, she looked at Iain and then at me, and with a small knowing smile she said, 'You pair of rascals.' She'd tasted the difference. She wanted us to know she hadn't lost her mind completely. Not yet.

The suction device Iain sometimes used to clear her windpipe began to terrorise her; she regarded it as one might an instrument of torture. The machine was noisy, and in her distorted condition, God knows what its roar suggested to her – some evil surgical implement, perhaps, intent on invading her body. She was drifting through a cloudscape of paranoia. Her lucid moments were quickly diminishing. She'd look into your face at times as if she'd never seen you before.

Once, when I was helping her change position on the bed – she couldn't do this on her own any more – I felt a hard lump the size of a pool-ball to the right of her lower spine. A new cancerous growth, another tumour, too late to do anything about it, the cancer was raging everywhere, it had spawned and spread, and spawned more and spread further, a lethal fungus. She was frail in my arms as I moved her, seventy pounds maybe, frangible as a plant in a season of drought. She gasped as I helped her lie down. The pink and red lights from the little Christmas tree gave the room a kind of sweet tranquillity that was only superficial; but she liked those lights. Occasionally she enjoyed listening to tapes of classical music on a cassette deck Stephen had placed in her room – but she was beginning to lose interest in music. *Shall I play something for you, Eileen?* She'd shake her head: *No*.

Sometimes, she'd rise suddenly from the bed, drawing strength from God knows what source, and rush out of the bedroom, dragging the oxygen tube behind her; panicky, she'd head towards the front door saying *I must get out of here, I must get out*, and then Nancy or Stephen or whoever else was present would lead her back to bed or make her sit on the sofa for a time until her anxiety had passed. These were bad moments, the worst. It was as if she thought that somewhere in the world there might be a destination in which she'd be safe from her disease, a place where she'd be healthy and free and mobile, if only she could find it. A paradise of vibrancy and well-being – and it lay tantalisingly beyond her reach.

A sense of death must have touched her at these times, the shadow of her dying must have crossed in front of her face and, frightened, she'd risen from her bed and tried to escape the presence in her bedroom. I didn't know. I was guessing. But this much was sure: the fear in her eyes came from that primal place where consciousness encounters the likelihood of its own demise, where you imagine yourself extinguished – and then what? Blackness and silence and nothing? Another world?

Eileen had always believed in the possibilities of a life after death; and perhaps other incarnations. Now she was scared – as if her belief system had just been blown away by the storm of impending death and lay around like the bits and pieces of an aeroplane shot out of the sky.

She no longer knew what was out there awaiting her.

I came to think of the living room as death's waiting room. We'd sit, in one or another combination of personnel, and listen for sounds from the bedroom where Eileen lay. We became adept at watching the open door of her bedroom, checking its glossy white surface for shadows that would mean she was on the move again. (The door had stickers Barbara had placed there whimsically on her last visit. One said OFFICE, the other MANAGER.)

We wanted Eileen to be still. We wanted her to be at peace. If she rose and slipped, she'd hurt herself. I'd see the Christmas tree lights reflected in the woodwork and hear the oxygen concentrator and sometimes the rattle of her coughing – at times a rasping, chilling sound that made you feel how powerless you were to help her.

One afternoon, she appeared in the living room. She walked in the kind of slow hesitant steps that suggest stiffness and pain; her balance was awkward. I hadn't heard her rise. She could move very quietly, surprisingly so, at times. I suggested she sit down, which she did. She stared at me; she seemed to be trying to place my face in her personal history.

'Campbell.' She said my name as recognition came to her.

And then she was quiet. Whether to break the silence that had fallen or whether to amuse her, I don't remember now, I sang the first couple of lines of *Danny Boy*. She covered her face with her hands and wept with a ferocity that was absolutely bewildering. I kneeled alongside her and took her hands and said, 'What is it? What's wrong?'

She whispered, 'That is such a beautiful song.'

And I understood; or I thought I did. She was having a moment of lucidity and knew she was leaving the world and all the things in it that delighted her – landscapes, sunsets, friends, her kids, the release of fragrance from a flower, song – and the first few phrases of that simple tune had reinforced this realisation. All the lights inside her were going out one by one; she knew she'd never hear that song again as surely as she knew she'd never read another book or sit on another beach at sunset with the sea singing or peel a tangerine for herself or cook another breakfast or hear a new piece of music or see her grandchildren grow up.

She knew. Yes, she knew.

Next morning she said she wanted to speak with me: she seemed very clear-headed. I lay beside her on the bed. She said, 'I haven't told anybody about this. Certain things are going on inside my body, Campbell. I know the signs are bad. And I've decided . . .' She'd hesitated, choosing her words with consideration. '. . . I'm not going to fight any more. The struggle's over.'

I heard myself weep. The shock of her words devastated me. I laid my head against her shoulder. She was saying goodbye.

I said, 'I'm sorry if I ever hurt you—'

She kissed me on the forehead and said, 'Ah, you loved me more than you ever hurt me.'

I was losing control: I felt all kinds of broken, choking sensations.

She said, 'You were the love of my life,' and her eyes fluttered closed.

I sat listening to her breathe but suddenly couldn't stay in the room. I had to go outside into that overbright, overblown Phoenix sunlight. I wanted to smoke and reached inside my shirt pocket for my cigarettes, but I'd given them up, I didn't have any. It didn't matter. I pressed my fingertips against the nicotine patch. I thought about what she'd said. *I was the love of her life.* I hadn't known that. I hadn't suspected it. The love of somebody's life – a great honour, an award I hadn't earned or deserved, a responsibility I hadn't shouldered very well.

I walked into the kitchen. Nancy Frick was loading the dishwasher. She saw how distraught I was. I heard myself say, 'I never meant to hurt her, Nancy. I never wanted to cause her any pain.'

'No, don't put yourself through this,' Nancy said. 'Let it go. Just let it go. We all do stuff we regret.' She laid a hand on my arm for a moment. I clutched the edge of the sink and shut my eyes and wished I could reach back and edit the past in such a way that nobody had ever been hurt and all our lives had been free of pain.

But none of this was a novel after all, and none of my flights of fancy could make it so. I had no control over the lives and fates of anyone. I couldn't make people healthy, except in books; and I couldn't impose happy endings on reality. I could try, of course I could, but my efforts were pointless in the end, puffs of wasted breath. No narrative strategy, no slick switches of location, no literary sleight of hand, no red herrings, no fresh dialogue could change anything in the situation. I thought about how I'd manipulated the lives of those closest to me, I'd dragged them here and there in the world at the

behest of my own whim. In search of what – my version of
reality? I'd flown them over oceans and continents, directed
them this way and that as if they were characters in a book
whose plot I'd devised. I thought of the long odyssey I'd
imposed on Eileen, from Glasgow to London to Brighton and
back to London and then to upstate New York and finally to
this desert, where she was to die; the journeys I'd forced on my
kids; and on Rebecca and Leda, from Arizona to Ireland.

Somewhere along the way either I had lost the storyline, or
Eileen's journey to death had shown me a new one: fiction was
where I hid.

The real world was where I lived.

Eileen never referred to our conversation again. Whether she
forgot it, whether it was a product of morphine, or whether she
simply preferred not to refer to it again, I didn't know. I only
knew that something almost indefinable had been settled
between us: there was forgiveness. But there always had been,
only now it was different, it was forgiveness with finality. If
there remained tiny vestigial grudges, ghosts of animosity, any
sediment of hurt – these were all gone.

The morphine tricked her, caused her delusions. Once, she
rushed from her bedroom trailing the oxygen tube, and headed
for the door leading to the patio. Iain stopped her.

'Where are you going, Mom?'

'To the fuzzy bus stop,' she said.

He led her back to her bedroom. Where in the world was
the fuzzy bus stop? In which disjointed reality did such a
thing belong? Iain was hurting; he hated this disease and how
it had afflicted his mother. But he saw a bleakly amusing side
to the effects of morphine on her. It was a small window out of
a grim situation, and although it didn't offer much in the way

of scenery, just the same it was a brief shift of perspective. Sometimes the answers she gave to his questions, or the remarks she made out of nowhere, caused him to smile in a sad way.

'Mom, do you know who I am?' he asked her once.

'Sure. You're the taxy-waxy man,' she answered.

The taxy-waxy man? The connections and constructs of her mind were just breaking down. I wondered if it was the morphine alone, or if the cancer had eaten into her brain now too.

Once, she told me she was going to the theatre, and I'd better hurry if I wanted to book tickets for our daughters. Daughters? She entered into a complicated halting explanation about seating arrangements, naming people I'd never heard of, daughters that had never existed; I couldn't follow any of it. Her train of thought was derailed. By now, she was hard to follow much of the time in any event, and the mind that had once been sharp, the instinct once so keen, were becoming blunted.

In Yorkshire, Barbara's health wasn't on an upward curve either; she discovered that the cancer was creating new growths in her large intestine, and there were further growths across her diaphragm, and the disease, as she put it so colourfully herself, 'has crept around two-thirds of my liver like a menacing oil-slick'. She began a course of hormone treatment and wasn't sure what the side effects might be. Despite her own life-threatening problems, she was unable to stop thinking about her mother. The phone calls were becoming impossible to take; the distance between herself and her mother was growing as Eileen faded.

On 19 January, Nancy telephoned from Phoenix and asked the question Barbara was asking herself. 'Is there any chance of you coming back to Phoenix? I hate to tell you this, Barb, but the Hospice nurses are saying Eileen hasn't got long . . . maybe a week, maybe a matter of days. Nobody's sure.'

So little time. Seven days. Six. Five. Who could predict the future? Cancer punched its own monstrous time-clock. 'I don't know how I can manage it, Nancy. I don't know how I'd raise the airfare, how my family would react . . .'

'I know, I know,' Nancy said. She added that a few days before, she'd taken Eileen out for a quick drive to pick up a mutual friend, Suzi, from the clinic. As Suzi climbed into Nancy's van, Eileen turned to Nancy and asked, 'Where's Barbara? I thought we were picking up Barbara?'

'No,' Nancy had said. 'Barbara is at home in England.'

With a forlorn expression, Eileen uttered the simple empty sound: 'Oh.'

When she heard this story, Barbara realised she had no choice; no matter how much the airfare cost, no matter that she was very ill herself, no matter that her time with her own family might be growing short, she'd return to Phoenix to see her mother before it was too late. If it wasn't already. She raised money in tiny amounts from friends; some of it came from Eileen's former colleagues at the clinic. She had enough for her ticket within the space of a day. She didn't have to explain anything to her family when it came to telling them; they'd been expecting her to go back one last time to her mother. They knew she couldn't stay away from Eileen.

She flew to Phoenix on 24 January, hoping all through the sleepless journey that there was enough life and spirit in Eileen to keep her alive long enough for them to see each other again. Nancy met her at Sky Harbor Airport.

'Am I too late?' Barbara voiced the question that had been gnawing at her relentlessly since she'd left Yorkshire.

Nancy hugged her and said, 'No, you're in time . . . but it doesn't look good, sweetie. It doesn't look good at all.'

On the night of 24 January, I met Barbara for the first time. Pale, stressed from sickness, she arrived at the apartment; she had only one destination in mind, her mother's bedroom. She had an unmistakable Yorkshire accent; she pronounced the word 'love' as 'loov', and 'must' became 'moost'. We barely had time to introduce ourselves to one another before she went to see Eileen, but I was struck by her presence, the keen questioning intelligence in her eyes (so similar to Eileen's), the little flashes of mischievous light that sometimes came into them. She had a gentle authority about her too. I liked her instantly. I admired the way she managed to put her own sickness to one side for the sake of her mother. I knew nothing at this time of the long search for Eileen, none of the details, the dead ends, the determination that had driven her. I was to learn all that.

She passed me, and went inside the bedroom. Eileen, saying nothing, tried to rise to greet her; her movements now were very slow. She managed to get herself into a sitting position on the edge of the bed, then Barbara helped her stand up, and wrapped her arms around her. And then she lay down again, patting the vacant side of the bed for Barbara to lie there alongside her.

Barbara rearranged the pillows – there were at least a dozen of them – and she climbed onto the bed. When Eileen was ready to settle, both women snuggled together, heads touching, legs resting against each other's and arms tightly clasped. Eileen kept whispering the same words, 'I love you, Barbara, I've missed you.' They fell asleep in a reassuring mother-child embrace.

When she woke later, Barbara was bothered by an aspect of the bedroom, something she couldn't get out of her mind. It was the smell, and it unsettled her, because she recognised it from her nursing days. It was the smell she associated with death.

Over the next few days, I was touched by the sincerity of the love Barbara showed towards her mother; she didn't want to leave her side. She was attached to her as if by magnetism. She stroked Eileen's face constantly and whispered to her, sang to her, or simply held her in prolonged silence. But she needed rest for her own sake; each night she'd go to Nancy's house, where she slept. Or tried to. But I knew she lay awake and worried about her mother. I knew she wasn't the kind of person who could simply pull the plug on her thoughts and anxieties and fall asleep.

She concerned me. She was driving herself hard. She was running on the raw energy of somebody who knows the death of a dearly loved one is near, that weird nervy dynamism fuelled by impending loss. Every second is a precious bonus. You're afraid you'll miss something if you go away. You have to stay close.

I had to urge her sometimes to leave the apartment. 'Go to Nancy's,' I'd say. We already had a degree of familiarity between us, because circumstance had thrown us into a hasty alliance. There wasn't time for the polite preliminary fencing that marks the opening of relationships; we'd been plunged into this one from the first meeting. But I knew we would have liked each other anyhow. She was straight, she saw into the heart of things, she had no time for elaboration or fuss; her speech was direct and her emotions didn't go through a labyrinth of filters before she could express them.

'For God's sake get some rest,' I'd tell her.

'I'm going, love, I'm going,' she'd say.

Sometimes she did, only to come back a few hours later.

*Mother's frailty*, she wrote, *is my main concern. She wants to move around all the time. It's as if she doesn't dare sit still for too long. Her movements are painfully slow. Walking a few steps, supported by people holding her hands, takes half an hour. And we have to make sure she's not left alone for a second.*

This awkward mobility of Eileen's, this urge to get up from her bed and shuffle pointlessly around the apartment, decreased in the days after Barbara's arrival. Now she could barely rise from her bed. By the time Keiron flew in from Seattle, she wasn't getting up at all, or if she did it was only with extreme reluctance.

Keiron took over the nightshift, and spent hours lying in bed beside his mother. He held her hand and talked to her constantly, ramblingly. He spoke of letting go. Of yielding. His patience astonished me. Where had he learned this gentleness? This . . . compassion?

My sons continued to amaze, even in their differences. Keiron and Stephen wanted their mother to go out quietly, as peacefully as possible; but Iain preferred to fight for her until the very end, because he'd been trained to maintain life and saw any other course of action as a betrayal of principle. This fundamental difference caused anger one night when I was in the apartment with the three boys.

Eileen was breathing with difficulty, and Iain wanted to go inside her bedroom and apply his plastic suction tube into her throat and vacuum the obstruction from her windpipe.

'Why?' I asked. 'What's the point, Iain?'

'Because she needs to be suctioned,' he said.

Like me, Stephen was against the idea. 'She's terrified of the noise that thing makes,' he said. 'It scares her more than it does her any good.'

'You don't know what you're talking about,' Iain said.

I said, 'How would it help anyway, Iain? Would it give her

another thirty seconds of life maybe? And what kind of life would it be? You wouldn't be doing her any favours.'

Iain was angered. He paused outside the door of Eileen's bedroom with his fists clenched and his face white. 'She needs to have it done,' he said. 'Don't you understand that? She needs to have it done!'

'No, she fucking well doesn't,' I said.

'Listen to her,' Iain said. 'How can you sit there and listen to that awful sound she's making?'

'We've *been* listening to her, Iain. And your little plastic device isn't going to make a damn bit of difference,' I said.

The atmosphere was charged. It seemed to me the kind of electric moment that contained an element of potential violence. It was an unhappy situation; a woman was dying, and her three sons and ex-husband were arguing in the next room about whether she should be left to die or if certain ministrations could prolong her life. Cancer created unworthy emotions, pointless conflicts, squalor in the heart.

Iain appeared grim and scared: he didn't want to lose his mother without trying one last time to help her the only way he knew how.

Keiron, the voice of reason, said, 'Hey, it's pointless to argue. We should leave her alone. Anyway we're all uptight. Chill.'

Iain said, 'I can help her, I know I can. But if you don't want me to, OK, fine, it's your problem. It's on your heads.'

Although he was enraged and frustrated, Iain relented. If he'd been alone, he'd have gone inside the bedroom with his suction machine.

We sat in silence for a while, and the tension seeped very slowly away. I saw how close attendance on the dying created imbalances; self-control was skin-deep, civility a veneer. We were all suffering. We were all furious with the direction of real events. Eileen's dying affected every one of us. We were all losing an essential part of our lives and our shared history. And yet that sense of loss was bringing us closer together than we'd been for a very long time; perhaps never.

Barbara spent as much time with Eileen as she could. She noticed how life drained from her mother in such a way that she could almost watch it leaving her, like a pale gas rising upwards and dispersing. Eileen could speak now only in the quietest of whispers, and if you wanted to hear what she was saying you had to bring your ear down to her mouth. But most of what she said was confusing.

My own moments with Eileen were usually silent ones now. Often she'd stare into the distance with that frightened look I'd seen before. She didn't want to give up this slender little hold she had on life, but she had no fight left. Her expression was one of almost constant distress.

Once, unexpectedly, she kissed me on the forehead and said, 'Help me.' I knew what she meant, I knew what she was asking for. As I'd done after her operation in hospital, I imagined holding a pillow over her face long enough for her to die. I imagined her raising a hand to clutch my wrist as the last of her life faded and a final darkness came down. I'd never sleep again; if I did, my dreams would be poisoned with turmoil and guilt. *Help me* – but I couldn't, not the way she wanted me to. I didn't have murder in my heart; nor euthanasia.

For some reason I started to describe a beach to her, the tide coming in and out on gleaming sands, gulls wheeling in the sky, seashells glistening under sunlight. Although she looked glazed and elsewhere, she was listening. I knew she was listening. I knew that in her mind she was walking on that beach and feeling the damp hard-packed sand under her bare feet as the shadows of gulls flickered across her face. I described this beach hour after hour, for so long in fact that when Rebecca came in and offered to relieve me I felt I was walking on the sands myself and a sun-warmed tide lapped my ankles, and I didn't want to get up, I didn't want to leave Eileen.

I said to Rebecca, 'I'll just stay a little longer.'

Rebecca went back inside the living room to sit with Iain. He sighed and gestured towards the bedroom where I held his mother's hand and talked on and on, like a man possessed, about the ocean and the white canvas sails of small boats and the unspoiled sands. I couldn't stop myself. On and on, the sea and the goddamn sand, the birds, the sun on water, what was wrong with me, was this some kind of breakdown, was the needle of the psyche stuck in the same groove, why didn't I want to leave this make-believe beach? I couldn't pull myself away, as long as I had the sea and the sand Eileen would be alive, as long as I didn't stop talking I would have her attention, and therefore her life wouldn't fade away . . . I was temporarily deranged, unhinged. My mind was filled with sky and the sound of tides. I caught myself. Throat dry, talked-out, I stopped. I was jangled and afraid: Eileen was going away from us. Nothing could keep her here in this world.

Rebecca told me later that while I'd been walking that beach with Eileen, Iain had smiled in a quiet way and, as if he were entrusting her with a great confidence, said: 'He's made up for all the bad times.'

On one occasion Eileen whispered to me, 'Tell this story.'

I must have looked befuddled.

'Tell this story,' she insisted. 'You know – of Barbara and me. How we found each other.'

I said I would. I promised I would.

\*

Barbara's experiences with her mother in the last days were usually the same as mine. Eileen would say 'Let me go' or 'Why can't I go?' Or, 'Help me to go.' The last words she ever said to Barbara were heart-rending: 'Please please, darling, put me to sleep.'

Eileen was slipping into another place. Her heart, Barbara noticed, was pounding visibly as the mechanism of her body struggled to survive, but her spirit was no longer present. Her eyes were open all the time, but empty. Barbara lay down beside her. She wrote, *I rest my head against hers and lovingly stroke her hand. I quietly sing her favourite song,* The Rose, *close to her ear. As I finish I become aware of a tear-drop on her face. It isn't mine.*

*I kiss her, knowing it's for the last time.*

*And I say goodbye.*

For almost two days Eileen lay with her blind eyes open; she didn't move, she simply stared into nothing. I sat beside her and held her hand for a time and I thought, *Please die, please be free, Eileen.* Whatever she was doing now, it wasn't living, it wasn't *close* to living. I didn't want to see her like this. None of us did. She was beyond the reach of help.

Early on the morning of 4 February, she died.

Thankfully, mercifully, she died.

Barbara went inside the bedroom where Eileen lay and had a private moment with her. She sat on the bed beside her and lifted her mother's lifeless hand into her own. The oxygen machine was silent now. There had been an unusually strong storm in the night, persistently heavy rain that had flooded the streets of the city. Barbara thought about how her mother had loved the rain, how she'd enjoyed the feel of it on her face. *It felt as though the storm had come to collect her,* she wrote, *as though she'd flown on the winds to her destination.* She stroked her mother's waxy lifeless hand and looked at her face, then she leaned over and kissed her cheek.

She said 'I love you,' and left the bedroom without looking back.

I waited until Barbara had gone before I stepped inside the room and looked at my ex-wife lying with her eyes still open and the pink-red lights of the tiny Christmas tree shining, and I went to her and, saying nothing because there was nobody to hear, simply touched the side of her cold face. I thought of our marriage and our life together and our children and the direction our lives had taken and how we'd split apart, and I felt sad in a way I'd never felt before, and yet relieved because I knew that, wherever she was, she was beyond any more hurt. And I thought too of the kindness and love she'd shown people in her life and I was glad her daughter had found her.

Nancy Frick handed me an envelope the day Eileen died. 'She wrote this for you last year,' she said. 'I was to give it to you after . . .' and she left the sentence unfinished.

I thanked Nancy and opened the envelope, which contained a letter Eileen had written to me on an unspecified day in November 1997. What could she say to me from beyond the grave? This is what she wrote:

*Dearest Campbell,*

*I am feeling it is getting near the time for me to leave. My body is giving me signals and I am experiencing a lot of pain. Living off aspirins is not my idea of quality life and I know the next step will be morphine. I do not relish a long drawn-out experience and it would be so hard on those around me. Of course, I could go rather quickly too, therefore I wanted to write to you while I can. Throughout the years I have always loved you. It seems to me deeper than a man/woman relationship. The best way I can describe it is at soul level. I think we were brought together because of what we had to offer each other at that level. If you had not divorced me, I may never have gone on to do what I have done with my life. You helped me to find myself and I am eternally grateful for that. You brought me to the States where I met my destiny, and you met Rebecca. Your mission was over, you had no need to stay in this country any more. For the 'bad' times I fully forgive you. I played my part too and hope you can forgive me. Between us, we brought into being three incredible sons. They have a deep love for both of us. I know you will be able to help them cope with my going on. I have cherished your friendship, Campbell. When you came here in July you literally gave me the strength to keep going. To have you there each day was a delight. To know that you cared so much was an even greater pleasure.*

*With everlasting love and appreciation, Eileen*

She was cremated on 5 February, her birthday.

The night before the memorial service, Barbara dreamed of her mother: *I'm standing in a room, and behind me in the corner my mum's lying dead in a bed. As I turn to look at her, she opens her eyes, starts breathing again. I sit by her side. Her features change. She becomes younger and younger, and her hair redder, longer. I watch as the process unfolds. It ends with her looking like a child of about twelve. She's taken me back to that time in her life when she'd been a happy, carefree child. It's a beautiful dream. I know she's in a better place now, but she'll always be very close. She's only round the corner, waiting for me.*

# Epilogue

I flick the pages of one of Eileen's old journals; it is a sunny day in Ireland, mid-August, 1998. Already the longest day of the year has passed, and the darkness will come sooner each evening, and then we'll be hurrying down towards winter, and turf-smoke from hearths will hang in the misty rain of villages. Summer is decaying. I think of this as I look through the pages of the journals – the relics of a life, the scribbled notes, the reminders Eileen made to herself. These are her aspirations, some of them unfulfilled, and her wishes, some of them not granted to her.

Here, for example, are her 'goals' for the period January to March 1994.

*Purchase new car by 28 Feb with loan from Credit Union*
*Begin exercise program – aerobics × 3 a week*
*Walk 2 miles × 2 a week*
*Pay off major credit cards by 31 March*

Did she walk two miles twice a week? Pay off her credit

cards? Join an aerobics class? I don't have answers; the questions are frozen on the pages of her notebooks.

There are pages of dream analysis, densely written; she jotted down her dreams immediately on waking, and spent hours interpreting their meanings and messages. She picked at them and probed them, until they yielded a truth or an instruction. There are other pages where she wrote out her fantasies about Peter, the married man; spending time with him, walking together in the woods, cooking dinner for him. There are fragments of unfinished letters to Peter; one contains the phrase 'men either leave me for other women, or will not leave other women for me'. I feel a stab of pain when I come across this; it's not because I am trespassing into her privacy, it's sorrow – and some hangover of remorse too, despite the fact she forgave me. But the truth is, I am a man who left her for somebody else. I belong in that clan.

She deserved better.


On my desk is the leaflet printed for the Memorial Service that took place in Phoenix on 6 February 1998. There's a brief biography of Eileen's life and career, and a short programme of events. The chapel was packed with people who'd come to say goodbye, including Leda, who'd flown in from Dublin just to attend the service. I was hugely surprised, because nobody had told me she was coming. A 12,000-mile round trip in only three days: Leda had stamina and resolve.

Nancy Frick rose to read the eulogy, which Rebecca had helped compose, but she was so overcome with emotion she couldn't speak. Instantly, Barbara got up from the front pew, picked up a red rose from the table where a collection of photographs of Eileen had been assembled, and stepped up to the podium to take over. Later, she'd think how uncharacteristic this was of her, because she didn't like appearing in front of a crowd, but at that moment she'd felt compelled to take Nancy's place.

A passage was read from 1 Corinthians: 12–13: this had been a favourite of Eileen's. *So faith, hope, love abide, these three; but the greatest of these is love.* I'd managed to locate a bagpiper the day before the service, and he played one of the most melancholy of Jacobite tunes, *The Skye Boat Song*. A solemn sound of home, so far away from Scotland, moved me as much as it moved everyone else in that chapel.

The boys wept; I saw Leda try to comfort them, especially Keiron. I wondered what images they'd have of their mother after this great outswelling of sadness had passed. Would Keiron remember his first guitar, a fifty-dollar Sunburst Harmony Eileen had bought him when he was about twelve and encouraged him to play? Would he remember her telling him that the most important lesson she could teach him in life was to be true to himself? And Stephen – what would come rushing back to him in moments of reflection? Would he remember how he'd made harmless fun of her near-sighted-ness, or the times when her mind was elsewhere and she'd call him Keiron or Iain, and not by his own name? Or how he didn't like going to a movie with her that she'd already seen, because she couldn't stop herself from saying *Now watch this bit coming up* or *Something's about to happen here you're not expecting*? Or would he always remember her appetite for life and the hours of her time she gave away like free gifts to others? And Iain – would he think of how happy she was when he telephoned her, and how he enjoyed their Sunday dinners and watching *60 Minutes* with her? Would he think how he'd lost his best friend – a blow so devastating to him that months later he'd find himself driving along and sud-denly remembering his mother and he'd yell angrily at God for putting her through such intense misery? And Barbara, who'd come back from the podium to sit between Keiron and Stephen and hold their hands, what was she thinking? She didn't have the same big memory-store to wander as the boys did; her time with her mother had been limited, but she was a part of this family too, and she had recollections of her own she'd never forget, memories of her search and its ultimate fulfilment, of deep love and great loss.

Suddenly I realised I was the only biological parent the boys had, and the thought – so obvious and yet so novel to me – filled me with a renewed sense of the significance of connections and, yes, of blood-ties. I remembered times when I'd thought about calling the boys, or sending them a quick e-mail, and how often I'd postponed these simple acts – the way I'd done with Eileen. I thought of time lost, time spilled and wasted. I resolved that there would be no more drift, no more gaps, that I'd build bigger and stronger bridges between us. We'd see each other more often. We'd communicate constantly. We'd make room for this. We wouldn't slide off into silences; we wouldn't be posted missing from one another.

I watched Stephen, strong and composed, even though his sorrow was enormous, go to the podium and read a short nonsense poem Eileen had written; it didn't mean anything. He explained: 'Mom just liked the sounds of the words.'

And then a period was set aside for anyone who felt a need to comment on Eileen. The first person who got up was Leda; in fact, she almost jumped up. She looked pale and delicate and a little nervous as she spoke about how Eileen had given her the most precious gift she could – a family. There was gratitude in her words, and sadness too; I was proud that she'd travelled so far to speak her feelings aloud. I was proud that day of all my children, the three sons I'd had with Eileen, the daughter I'd inherited when Rebecca came into my life.

We were family. We'd come together. And it had taken tragedy to create this fusion.

Dennis Morton, returned from Santa Cruz, also paid tribute to Eileen, but he was overcome in much the same way as Nancy had been. Others got up, talked, reminisced, laughed at good memories, funny stories; but it's in the nature of these gatherings that sorrow isn't far away. A man called Stapleton, whom I'd never seen before, came to the podium to express his gratitude, in a voice very close to tears, for the way Eileen had helped him deal with the death of his daughter.

He began to tell a story of his time in Vietnam – *Vietnam?* I wondered where he was going with this narrative, and what part an old war played in Eileen's life: grainy newsreel images went through my head, burning oil blackening skies and naked children fleeing napalmed villages. Stapleton spoke of how he'd carried a wounded soldier towards a waiting helicopter, and along the way he'd encountered an American GI dying of his wounds.

The dying man had a flak jacket he offered to Stapleton with the words, 'Your buddy needs this more than me. Take it.'

Stapleton took the jacket and wrapped it around his injured companion and continued towards the chopper. He never learned the name of the dying GI. He knew only this: faced with his own death, the soldier had acted with selfless humanity. His last act may have been the finest of his life; who would ever know?

And this was the parallel Stapleton was drawing between Eileen and an event in Vietnam more than twenty years before. He'd tried to phone her while she was on her deathbed, because he was still depressed about his daughter, but she'd been too sick to come to the telephone. A few days later, it seemed, she'd somehow found the strength to return his call.

Nobody knew she'd done this, not Nancy, not me, not Stephen. She must have called him back in a secret moment because she cared about his shaky state of mind – and God knows where she found the courage to comfort somebody else in the face of her own dying. The living, I thought, don't have a monopoly on surprises; the dead can spring them too.

The service ended with Eileen's favourite popular song: *The Rose*.

In March, Stephen brought Eileen's ashes to Ireland from Phoenix. I travelled with him to Yorkshire where we collected Barbara; Stephen met Heidi again, and was introduced to Nick and Barbara's two sons for the first time. He took pleasure in the fact that they called him Uncle Stephen, and appeared to hold him in esteem – he was the friendly young uncle who'd travelled all the way from exotic Arizona to this corner of Yorkshire.

We left England – Barbara, Stephen and myself – and we drove north to Scotland on a day of blistering black rain and dirty spray kicked up by the wheels of big trucks on the motorway. In Glasgow, we went to a park in the southern part of the city, close to where Eileen had been born and brought up. This park was special to her, normally a place of tranquillity; and it was special to me too, weighted as it was with memories of Eileen and me walking together beneath these trees, hand in hand, in love. Neither of us could have foreseen that we'd return here on death's sad business.

Rain hammered violently against the surface of a pond and streams sputtered angrily down a steep incline in the earth. I watched Barbara and Stephen take the container of ashes and scatter them to the weather and saw how the white powder was tugged by the wet wind and blown to the sodden ground.

Then Stephen and Barbara threw some rose petals, saved

from the memorial service, over the ashes. After that, they held one another for a time as the rain hit the earth with the force of nails. I felt sad, but good on some deeper level: Eileen was home. And one of the people who'd brought her home was the daughter she'd given away.

Barbara keeps souvenirs of her mother at her house in Yorkshire. A ring Eileen had presented her with on their first meeting; a necklace, originally given to Eileen by Keiron as a gift (Barbara wears it constantly); photographs of Eileen and the boys on the bedside table; dried rose petals in a vase on the window ledge – red from the memorial service, mixed with yellow, because yellow was Eileen's favourite colour; Eileen's battered old gardening hat, a scarf, a few items of her clothing.

*Strange,* Barbara wrote to me in August 1998, *this time last year I had no idea who my mother was, where she was, whether she was alive or dead, if I would ever find her and meet her. And now I have photographs of her in my bedroom and I wear her jewellery, and I have hundreds of wonderful memories.*

Eileen once said to Barbara: 'It doesn't feel right that we found each other just to die. It doesn't make sense.' But Barbara has made sense of it: 'What she and I experienced in four months was far more intense and valuable than many mothers and daughters experience in a lifetime. I am profoundly grateful for it.'

I think of Barbara now. I think of her fighting her disease, the dignity and resilience she brings to the struggle. She has good days and bad. She has become a communications centre in our lives: the boys telephone her or send her letters, and sometimes, when she isn't breaking a confidence, she may forward these notes to me. She's the switchboard. She's HQ. She's Central Office. Keiron is planning a trip to see her in

Yorkshire. He and Stephen are in touch with her all the time. They tell her things they don't tell me. She knows more about the state of Stephen's marriage than I do. In a way, she's replaced Eileen in the lives of the boys: Big Sister becomes Mother. Iain, grappling with the mysteries of organic chemistry at school, writes to her whenever the pressure of his studies permits.

No day passes without at least one note from her to me, which usually begins with the question: *is anybody there?* And if I don't hear from her, I worry – is she OK? Is she in too much pain to go to her computer? And then a message will come through: *is anybody there?* And I'll feel a surge of relief that this link with Eileen is still vibrant, that a very important part of Eileen is still with us.

I want Barbara always to be there, sending her messages.

In early April, two months after she'd died, I had a dream that Eileen was sitting, hunched and ill, on the edge of our bed. Rebecca was fast asleep. Eileen, dressed entirely in white, beckoned for me to follow her out of the bedroom and down the long corridor to my office.

It was a realistic dream, hauntingly so. Her finger was crooked, and she was persistent; she was telling me that I had a book to write, I'd made a promise, I had to keep it.

I'd like the impossible now: I'd like her to read the book. But she's gone. And unless she comes back again in the dead of some other night, I have no way of telling her that this time I kept my word.

Or maybe she knows.

# Postscript

Barbara died on July 5, 1999. Shortly before her death, she was able to read the finished manuscript of this book, and make certain corrections to the text. She had a copy of the book-jacket on her bedside table, and a photograph of her mother.